HEALTHY BACK
ANATOMY

General Disclaimer

The contents of this book are intended to provide useful information to the general public. All materials, including texts, graphics, and images, are for informational purposes only and are not a substitute for medical diagnosis, advice, or treatment for specific medical conditions. All readers should seek expert medical care and consult their own physicians before commencing any exercise program or for any general or specific health issues. The author and publishers do not recommend or endorse specific treatments, procedures, advice, or other information found in this book and specifically disclaim all responsibility for any and all liability, loss, or risk, personal or otherwise, which is incurred as a consequence, directly or indirectly, of the use or application of any of the material in this publication.

Thunder Bay Press
An imprint of Printers Row Publishing Group
10350 Barnes Canyon Road, Suite 100, San Diego, CA 92121
www.thunderbaybooks.com

North American Compilation Copyright © 2010, Thunder Bay Press
Copyright © 2010 by Moseley Road Inc.

Printers Row Publishing Group is a division of Readerlink Distribution Services, LLC.
Thunder Bay Press is a registered trademark of Readerlink Distribution Services, LLC.

All notations of errors or omissions should be addressed to Thunder Bay Press, Editorial Department, at the above address. All other correspondence (author inquiries, permissions) concerning the content of this book should be addressed to Moseley Road, Inc., 123 Main Street, Irvington, NY 10533. www.moseleyroad.com.

Thunder Bay Press
Publisher: Peter Norton
Associate Publisher: Ana Parker
Publishing Team: April Farr, Kelly Larsen, Kathryn C. Dalby
Editorial Team: JoAnn Padgett, Melinda Allman, Dan Mansfield
Production Team: Jonathan Lopes, Rusty von Dyl

ISBN: 978-1-68412-088-8

Printed in China

22 21 20 19 18   2 3 4 5 6

HEALTHY BACK
ANATOMY

A Chiropractor's Guide to a Pain-Free Back

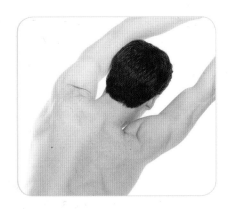

Philip Striano, DC

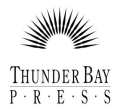

THUNDER BAY
P·R·E·S·S

San Diego, California

CONTENTS

HEALTHY BACK BASICS

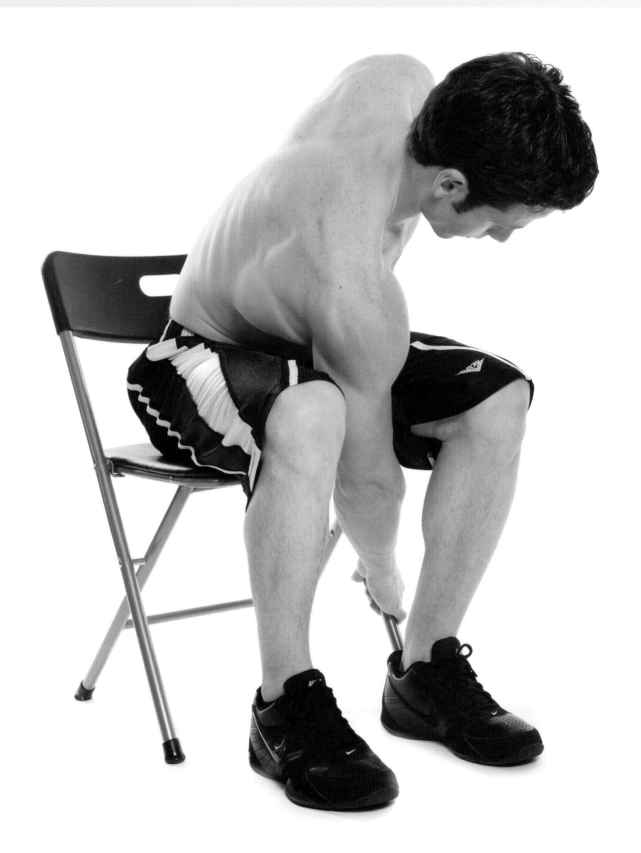

Lower-back and neck pain are some of the most common health problems in adults today. They are the second-most prevalent reason for doctors' visits, especially lower-back pain. With society having an increasingly older population and people living more sedentary lifestyles, back and neck pain are sure to afflict more people in the future than they ever have in the past.

There are many contributing risk factors to back and neck pain. A partial list of these factors includes age, obesity, physical activity (both too little and too much), poor posture, psychological stress, trauma, and poor work ergonomics.

Through awareness, action, and education, however, you can decrease your susceptibility to neck and lower-back pain. Make yourself aware of the potentially harmful factors in your lifestyle. Be cognizant of your overall health. Your body is constantly talking to you—listen to it. Pain and fatigue are two of the warning signs your body will send you. Take action, eat, rest, play, and exercise properly. Finally, educate yourself on how to do these things the right way and in the right amount.

This book is written to give a generally healthy person the tools to prevent chronic back and neck pain. If you currently suffer from a serious back or neck injury, please consult with your physician before starting a stretching or strengthening program.

It is of prime importance to make sure that you warm up your body before doing any of the stretches or strengthening exercises. You do not want to stretch a cold or stagnant muscle—this can lead to tearing of the muscle fibers. Running or walking for a few minutes, or even a hot shower or bath, will warm up your muscles before exercise. This will increase blood flow, lubricate your joints, and prepare you for a safe exercise regimen. Make sure to drink plenty of water, around sixty-four ounces per day. This will prevent dehydration and allow your body to excrete toxins that it will be breaking down during exercise.

In the event that you do injure yourself, do not put heat on the injured area. Use ice on the injured area for the first forty-eight hours post-injury. To apply ice properly, leave on the injured area for twenty minutes, then take it off for an hour, and repeat. You can repeat multiple times throughout the day. The purpose of the ice is to decrease inflammation. If the ice is left on for more than twenty minutes, you will get a reverse reaction and your body will bring fluid into the area, increasing inflammation and worsening the injury. If you ice properly and immediately after an injury, you can greatly reduce the duration and intensity of the injury. After the first two days, you can introduce heat to the affected area. It is also advisable to seek a doctor's opinion if you believe the injury warrants it.

ANATOMY OF A HEALTHY SPINE

Your spine is a well-crafted feat of anatomical engineering, forming your body's main upright support and allowing you to bend forward, backward, and sideways, as well as to twist and rotate. The spinal column also protects the spinal cord, which is the main pathway of the nervous system.

The Vertebrae

Twenty-four bones, called vertebrae, are stacked in a column to make up the spine. The spine is divided into three regions: the cervical vertebrae, the thoracic vertebrae, and the lumbar vertebrae. The cervical vertebrae are the seven vertebrae of the neck. They are known as C1 through C7. The topmost cervical vertebra, called the atlas, supports your skull. The twelve vertebrae of the upper and middle back, the thoracic vertebrae, are called T1 through T12. The vertebrae of the lower back, the lumbar vertebrae, are known as L1 through L5. The L5, the lowest vertebrae, connects to the top of the sacrum, which is a triangular bone at the base of the spine that fits between the two pelvic bones. At the base of the sacrum, at the very bottom of the spine, is the coccyx, or tailbone.

In each of the vertebrae (except for the atlas), a large, round, flat area called the vertebral body makes up the bulk of the bony structure. Attached to the back of each vertebral body is a bony, triangular ring, which is made up of two kinds of bones: two pedicle bones connect directly to the back of the vertebral body, and two lamina bones form the outer rim of the bony ring. Where the lamina bones join is a bony projection called the spinous process, which is the pointy bone that you can feel and see at the back of your spine. Two bony knobs, called the transverse processes, also jut from the sides of each vertebra. Because the vertebrae are stacked in a column, the bony ring forms a tube that allows your spinal cord to pass through, while protecting it on all sides.

A joint, known as the facet joint, connects each adjacent vertebrae to the one below it. The facet joints are the key links in the spinal chain, allowing the spine to move. Along with the facet joints, thin ligaments that run the length of the spine, as well as smaller ligaments, bind the vertebrae together. A number of muscles attach to the vertebra, controlling the movements of the spine.

vertebral body (with disk sitting on top)

transverse processes

spinal cord

spinous process

facet joints

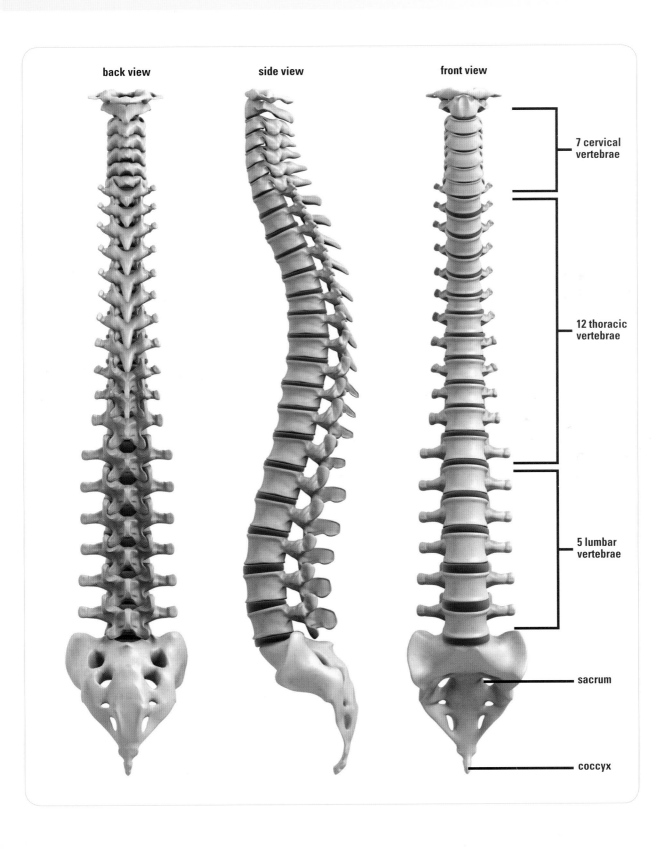

back view

side view

front view

7 cervical vertebrae

12 thoracic vertebrae

5 lumbar vertebrae

sacrum

coccyx

SPINAL CURVES

When you take a look at a healthy back from the side, you can see that the spine curves. The thoracic spine should curve slighty outward. The outward curve is called kyphosis. The cervical and lumbar spine both have a slight inward curve called lordosis. Both terms—*kyphosis* and *lordosis*—are often used to describe abnormally excessive curvatures of the spine

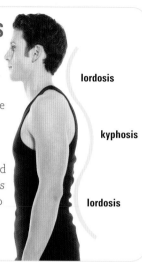

lordosis

kyphosis

lordosis

To add further stability to the spinal column, the twenty-four costae, or rib bones, attach directly to the thoracic spine, twelve on each side. All but the bottommost rib on each side also attach to the sternum, or breastbone, at the front of the chest.

The Spinal Disks

Separating each vertebra is an intervertebral disk that sits on top of the vertebral body and acts as a cushion between the bones. Rings of different kinds of tissue make up this shock-absorbing disk. Outermost is the annulus, which is composed of strong, elastic tissue called cartilage. The middle of the disk, the nucleus, is a slightly softer area. When you are young, the nucleus contains plenty of water, but as you age, it normally contains less water and begins to flatten.

The Nerves

Within the hollow tube formed by the interconnected vertebrae lies the spinal cord, which extends from the brain to the L2 vertebra. The spinal cord is like a long, branching wire made up of millions of nerve fibers that transmit neural signals between the brain and the body. The spinal cord is the conduit for motor and sensory information, and it also coordinates certain reflexes.

Nerves pass through each vertebra via small tunnels on both sides called the neural foramina. The nerves of the lumbar spine, called the cauda equina, go to the pelvic organs and lower limbs.

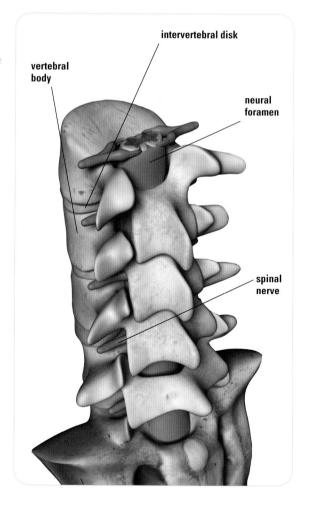

vertebral body

intervertebral disk

neural foramen

spinal nerve

THE MAJOR MUSCLES OF THE BACK

The most important task of the back muscles is to limit and control back motion and support the spine. While doing that, they also allow you to move, bend, twist, and stretch. There are three major muscle groups: the superficial muscles that act on the upper limbs, the intermediate muscles of the thorax, and the deep muscles of the vertebral column.

The Superficial Layer

The superficial layer of muscles are those that lie just beneath the skin. There are five pairs of muscles in the superficial layer: the latissimus dorsi, the trapezius, the rhomboideus major and minor, and the levator scapulae.

The latissimus dorsi muscles are the widest and most powerful of the back muscles, located one on each side. These triangular muscles help you extend, rotate, and pull your arms toward your body.

Together the two trapezius muscles that span the neck, shoulders, and back resemble a trapezoid, or diamond-shaped quadrilateral. These muscles move the scapula in a number of different ways, and allow movements like the shrug, in which the shoulders are lifted up in a straight line. The trapezius muscles also help rotate the head and neck and support the weight of the arms. They also help open up the chest for breathing.

The rhomboids (major and minor), also known as the "posture" muscles, lie between the scapulae and aid in rotation, elevation, and retraction of the scapulae.

The levator scapulae muscles extend along the back of the neck. These muscles elevate the scapulae and assist the functioning of various neck, arm, and shoulder movements.

The Intermediate Layer

Lying beneath the superficial layer of muscles is the intermediate layer that consists

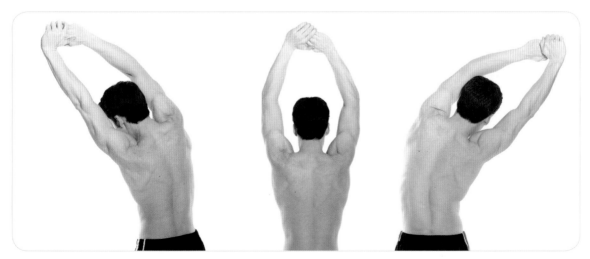

In a healthy back, a complex group of muscles work in harmony to support the spine and help hold the body upright. This large group also allows the torso to move, twist, and bend in many directions.

THE MAJOR MUSCLES OF THE BACK

of two muscles that act on the ribs. These pairs of muscles are the serratus posterior superior and the serratus posterior inferior. The serratus posterior superior raises the ribs to which it attaches. This movement expands the chest and aids respiration. The serratus posterior inferior draws the lower ribs backward and downward.

The Deep Layer

The muscles lying in the deep layer are the hardworking ones responsible for keeping you in an erect position, whether you are sitting or standing. These deep muscles include the erector spinae group and the splenius capitis.

The erector spinae is really not just one muscle but paired bundles of muscles and tendons that run more or less vertically in the grooves at each side of the vertebral column. The erector spinae muscles extend throughout the lumbar, thoracic, and cervical regions. This amazingly strong group functions to straighten the back and to rotate it sideways.

The splenius capitis muscles are a pair of broad, straplike muscles in the back of the neck. These muscles allow you to rotate and move your head.

Other Muscles

A healthy back relies on other muscles to function properly, including the muscles of the chest, abdomen, and lower body.

Intimately related to the back muscles are those of the shoulders. The deltoid muscles, divided into the deltoideus anterior, medialis, and posterior, form the outer layer of the shoulder muscles. Along with the deltoids are a group of muscles that stabilize the shoulder, known collectively as the rotator cuff. The rotator cuff is made up of the infraspinatus, subscapularis, supraspinatus, and teres minor.

The core muscles of the chest and abdomen, such as the pectorals, help increase our range of movement and serve an essential purpose to our everyday lives. The abdominal muscles, the rectus abdominis and transversus abdominis, are a series of muscles located on the lower midsection of the torso that contract the body forward. The side abdominal muscles, the obliquus externus and internus, are located on each side of the rectus abdominis. These muscles are involved in flexing the rib cage and the pelvic bones together, sideward bending of the torso, and rotation of the torso.

The major leg muscles can be broken down into three groups: the quadriceps femoris, the hamstrings, and the calf muscles. The quadriceps femoris consists of the major muscles of the front thigh—the vastus lateralis, vastus medialis, vastus intermedius, and rectus femoris. These knee extensor muscles allow us to walk, run, jump, and squat. The hamstrings are the muscles of the back thigh—the semitendinosus, semimembranosus, and biceps femoris. The hamstrings act upon both the hip and knee joints. Like the quads, this group of muscles is crucial to our ability to walk, run, and jump.

The major muscles of the calf are the gastrocnemius and the soleus. Both work to raise the heel.

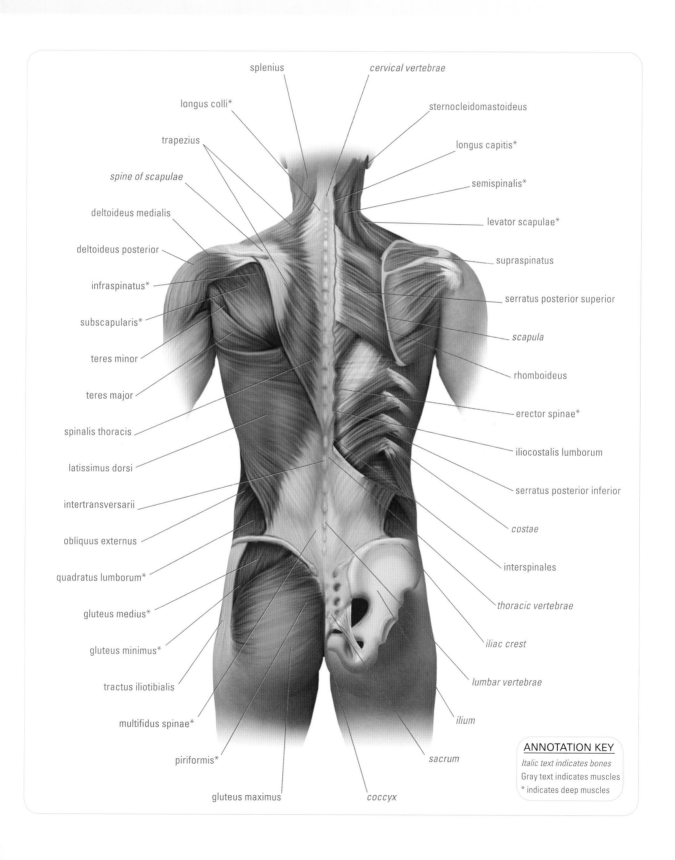

splenius

cervical vertebrae

longus colli*

sternocleidomastoideus

trapezius

longus capitis*

spine of scapulae

semispinalis*

deltoideus medialis

levator scapulae*

deltoideus posterior

supraspinatus

infraspinatus*

serratus posterior superior

subscapularis*

scapula

teres minor

rhomboideus

teres major

erector spinae*

spinalis thoracis

iliocostalis lumborum

latissimus dorsi

serratus posterior inferior

intertransversarii

costae

obliquus externus

interspinales

quadratus lumborum*

thoracic vertebrae

gluteus medius*

iliac crest

gluteus minimus*

lumbar vertebrae

tractus iliotibialis

ilium

multifidus spinae*

piriformis*

sacrum

gluteus maximus

coccyx

ANNOTATION KEY
Italic text indicates bones
Gray text indicates muscles
* indicates deep muscles

BACK PAIN

Your back is an amazing collection of bones, ligaments, tendons, muscles, and nerves, put together so as to be incredibly strong and highly flexible. Still, as with any complex structure, problems can arise, causing the all-too-common back pain so many of us suffer.

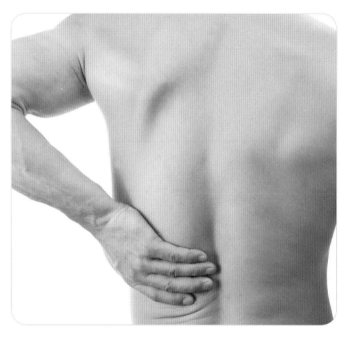

Finding the Cause

Back pain finds its roots in a variety of causes, and it can originate in any one of the back's components. Irritation of the large nerve roots that travel to the legs and arms causes back pain, as does irritation of the smaller spinal nerves. Straining the muscles or injuring the bones and ligaments of the back also results in pain. And for many, the intervertebral disks and the spaces between them are a source of pain.

Cervical Pain

Cervical, or neck, pain is usually caused by a muscle, ligament, or tendon strain. Most neck pain caused by strain will usually heal with time and nonsurgical treatments, but certain cervical problems may need more intensive treatment. For example, a cervical herniated disk produces pain that radiates down the arm, as does foraminal stenosis, a narrowing of the spinal foramen, pinching a nerve in the neck. Treatment options for neck pain will differ depending on the specific diagnosis.

Thoracic Pain

The twelve vertebral bodies of the thoracic spine are firmly attached to the rib cage and provide stability and structural support to the upper back, while allowing very little motion. The lack of motion in the thoracic area of the spine means that injuries to this area are rare. Nonetheless, a strain or irritation to the large muscles of the upper and mid back can produce quite severe back pain.

Lumbar Pain

The lumbar spine's wide range of motion, along with its role as weight bearer for the torso, means that it is far more prone to injury that the thoracic spine. In fact, half of the back's flexion, or forward bending, occurs at the hips, and the other half occurs at the lower spine, with most of that occurring at the L4–L5 and L3–L4 segments. With all this wear and tear, it is no wonder that these are the areas that most often break down—and cause pain. The wide range of movement also means the two lowest disks (L4–L5 and L5–S1) take a beating, resulting in a greater chance of herniation. A herniated disk can cause lower-back pain and often numbness that radiates through the leg and down to the foot. This condition is known as sciatica.

The biggest culprit in lower-back pain, however, is muscle strain. Like cervical strain, however, these areas will often heal with time and nonsurgical treatments.

Vertebral Compression

Trauma can cause a vertebral compression fracture, but it takes quite a severe trauma to break the bones of the spine. The vertebral bodies of your spine are built to support weight, but bones weakened by age or conditions such as osteoporosis are prone to developing compression fractures, and in severe cases can break with little or no force. The most common site of compression fractures is the lower back. These fractures can lead to chronic back pain and progressive spinal misalignment or deformity.

Disk Degeneration

As we age, the spinal disks dehydrate and stiffen, which makes it harder for them to adjust to compression. For some individuals, this natural aging process can cause chronic or acute pain.

Sacral Pain

Below the lumbar spine is the sacrum, the bone that makes up the back part of the pelvis. Connecting the sacrum to the iliac bones of the pelvis are the sacroiliac joints. Pain in the sacrum often originates from sacroiliac joint dysfunction. Sacroiliac pain is more common in men than in women.

Muscle and Ligament Pain

The two most common causes of back pain are muscle strains and ligament sprains. But what is the difference between a strain and a sprain? When you abnormally stretch or tear a muscle, that is a strain. When you tear ligaments (the tough, fibrous bands of tissue that hold bones together) from their attachments, that is a sprain. Although the causes are different, both produce similar symptoms: pain and muscle spasms. These symptoms result from the inflammation of soft tissue that results from either a strain or sprain. Because the lumbar spine is engaged in almost all movement, lumbar muscle strains and sprains are the most common back complaints.

PRESSURED AND PINCHED NERVES

Because an intervertebral disk sits directly in front of each neural foramen, a bulged or herniated disk can narrow the opening—thus putting pressure on the nerve and causing pain.

At the back of the foramen sits a facet joint. Facet joints can form bone spurs; a bone spur can project into the tunnel, narrowing the hole and painfully pinching the nerve.

EXERCISING FOR A HEALTHY BACK:

Professor Vladimir Janda was a Czechoslovakian-born neurologist and physiatrist, and a renowned practitioner and lecturer in the area of musculoskeletal health care. Janda's teachings are accepted and practiced by chiropractors, physical therapists, osteopaths, and medical doctors throughout the world today.

Janda's observations and research led to his discovery of predictable patterns of muscular imbalances throughout the body. He named these imbalances the upper-crossed and lower-crossed syndromes. In short, Janda noticed that prolonged static postural positions, such as sitting in a chair all day long or sleeping with multiple pillows under your head, lead to predictable muscle patterns. When a muscle is in a facilitated, or tight, state for an extended period, it will reflexively lead to an inhibition, or weakening, of muscles on the opposite side of the body. This pattern is called reciprocal inhibition, in which the normal movement patterns of your body become aberrant and your muscles work out of sequence. This leads to muscles and joints taking on more work and greater stress, which culminates in joint pain and myofascial, or soft-tissue, pain.

Upper-crossed and lower-crossed syndromes are most commonly found in people with chronic conditions, with problems that have existed for more than eight weeks. In order to correct these imbalances, you need to identify tight muscles and stretch them, and also work to strengthen the corresponding weak muscles. Exercising in this way will lead the body to better balance, or homeostasis, allowing for the proper recruitment pattern of muscles to do ordinary movements. In turn, this will reduce myofascial pain and unnecessary stress and early degeneration of the joints.

Many things can cause chronic muscular imbalances, including poor posture, overuse of muscles, joint dysfunction, poor repetitive biomechanics, trauma, and psychological stress. To eliminate the imbalances, you must identify the contributing factors, and then seek treatment and an exercise regimen from appropriate health-care practitioners. You can stretch and strengthen the appropriate muscles properly, but if the provocative agent is not removed, the patterns are destined to repeat themselves.

EXERCISE AIDS

A few simple props can help you get the most from your exercise regimen, such as small hand weights, medicine balls, and a Swiss ball.

A Swiss ball, which is shown in many of the following exercises, is a large, heavy-duty inflatable ball, ranging in diameter from 18 to 30 inches. The ball is unstable, and you have to constantly adjust your balance while performing a movement, which helps you improve your balance, proprioception, and flexibility.

Swiss balls were originally developed for use by physical therapy and chiropractic patients, but they are now regular aids in many fitness regimens, including yoga and core training. Swiss balls come in a range of sizes, so if you purchase one, be sure to take into consideration your individual weight and height.

THE JANDA APPROACH

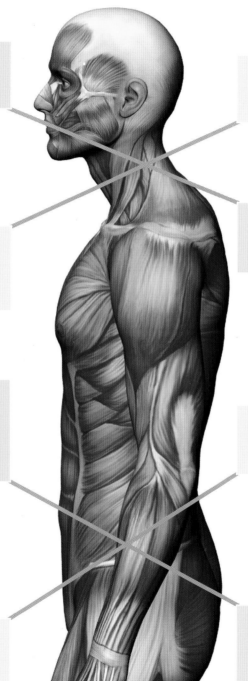

UPPER-CROSSED SYNDROME

INHIBITED
- longus capitis
- longus colli

FACILITATED
- sternocleidomastoideus
- pectoralis major
- pectoralis minor

FACILITATED
- upper trapezius
- levator scapulae

INHIBITED
- lower trapezius
- levator scapulae

LOWER-CROSSED SYNDROME

INHIBITED
- rectus abdominis
- transversus abdominis
- obliquus externus
- obliquus internus

FACILITATED
- rectus femoris
- iliopsoas

FACILITATED
- thoracolumbar extensors

INHIBITED
- gluteus maximus
- gluteus medialis
- gluteus minimus

FULL-BODY ANATOMY

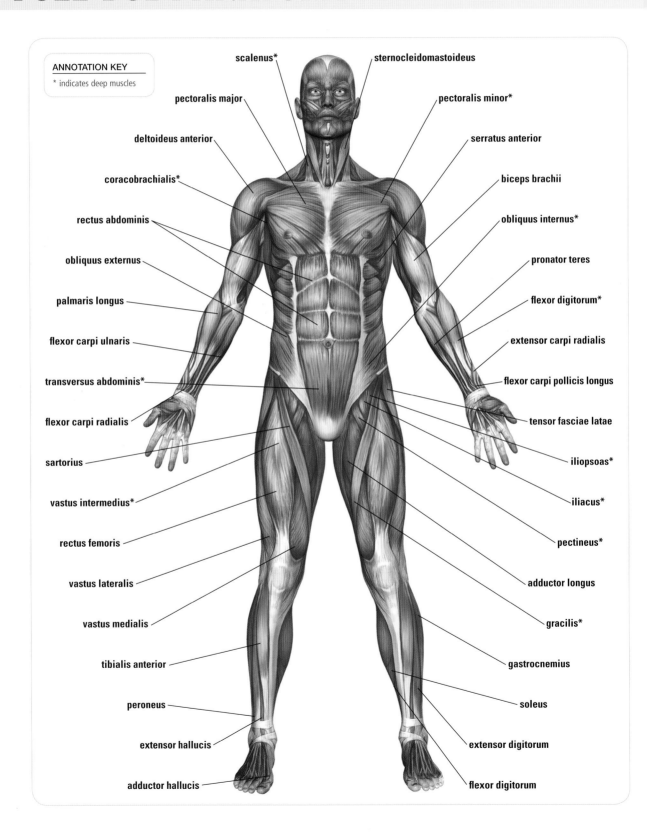

ANNOTATION KEY

* indicates deep muscles

scalenus*

sternocleidomastoideus

pectoralis major

pectoralis minor*

deltoideus anterior

serratus anterior

coracobrachialis*

biceps brachii

rectus abdominis

obliquus internus*

obliquus externus

pronator teres

palmaris longus

flexor digitorum*

flexor carpi ulnaris

extensor carpi radialis

transversus abdominis*

flexor carpi pollicis longus

flexor carpi radialis

tensor fasciae latae

sartorius

iliopsoas*

vastus intermedius*

iliacus*

rectus femoris

pectineus*

vastus lateralis

adductor longus

vastus medialis

gracilis*

tibialis anterior

gastrocnemius

peroneus

soleus

extensor hallucis

extensor digitorum

adductor hallucis

flexor digitorum

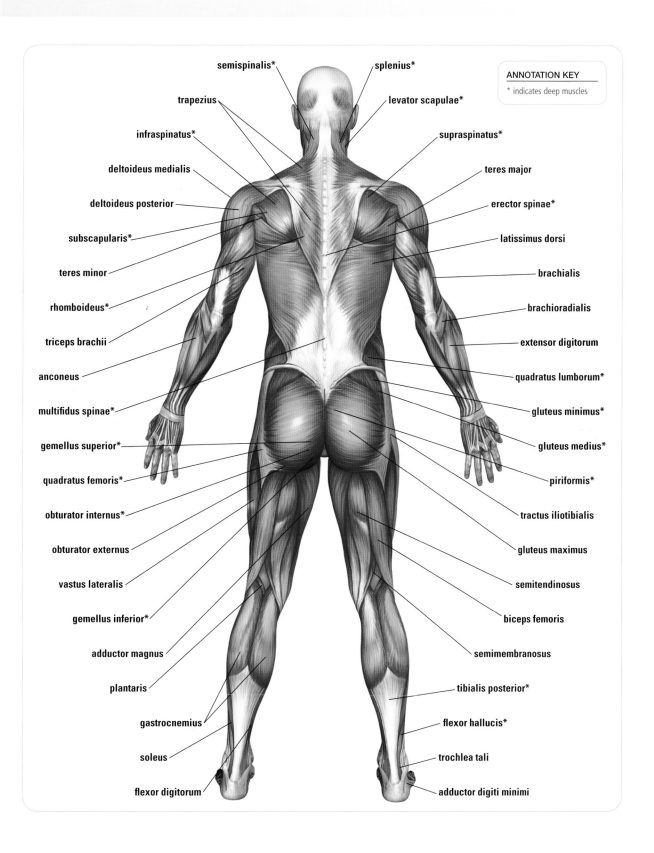

ANNOTATION KEY
* indicates deep muscles

semispinalis*
splenius*
trapezius
levator scapulae*
infraspinatus*
supraspinatus*
deltoideus medialis
teres major
deltoideus posterior
erector spinae*
subscapularis*
latissimus dorsi
teres minor
brachialis
rhomboideus*
brachioradialis
triceps brachii
extensor digitorum
anconeus
quadratus lumborum*
multifidus spinae*
gluteus minimus*
gemellus superior*
gluteus medius*
quadratus femoris*
piriformis*
obturator internus*
tractus iliotibialis
obturator externus
gluteus maximus
vastus lateralis
semitendinosus
gemellus inferior*
biceps femoris
adductor magnus
semimembranosus
plantaris
tibialis posterior*
gastrocnemius
flexor hallucis*
soleus
trochlea tali
flexor digitorum
adductor digiti minimi

CERVICAL EXERCISES

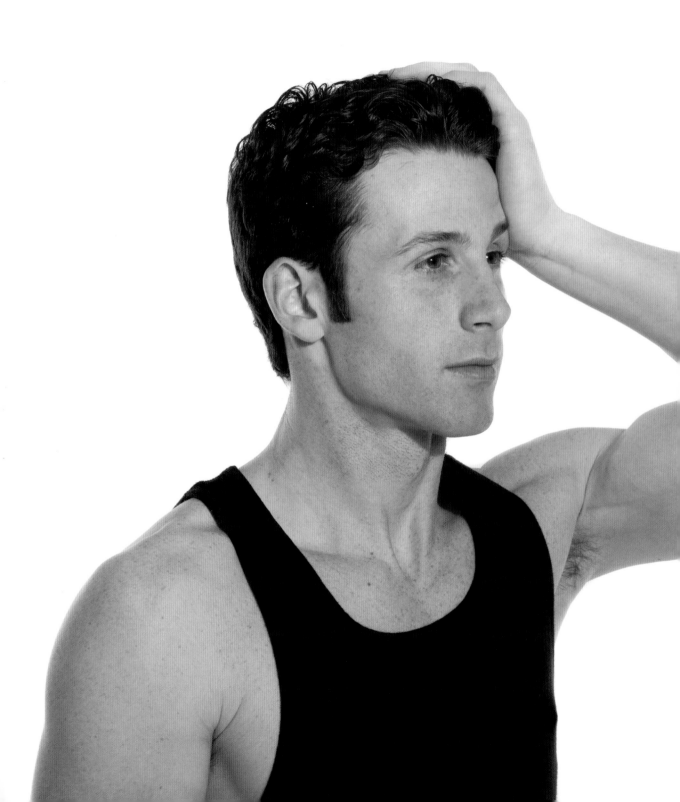

Although most neck pain isn't serious, it's a common complaint among adults. From spending hours hunched in front of our computers to slumping on the sofa to watch TV, many of us suffer from the effects of poor posture. Sprains and injuries, as well as ailments such as arthritis or pinched nerves, also result in neck pain and/or compromised range of motion.

A healthy back starts with a healthy neck, so it makes sense that cervical spine exercises are key components of a healthy back regimen. Many of the following exercises appear to be quite simple, but if performed correctly they can strengthen your cervical spine and keep your neck flexible and mobile. Getting the neck moving is essential for relieving all-too-prevalent neck pain or stiffness, but keep in mind that good form is a must. Perform the following exercises slowly and carefully—you want to feel a stretch, not pain.

FLEXION STRETCH

CERVICAL

1 Sit or stand, keeping your neck, shoulders, and torso straight. Place one or both hands behind your head.

2 Slowly pull your chin toward your chest until you feel a stretch in the back of your neck.

3 Hold for ten seconds, and repeat three times.

ANNOTATION KEY
Italic text indicates ligaments
Bold text indicates active muscles
Gray text indicates stabilizing muscles
* indicates deep muscles

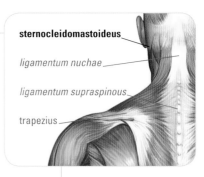

sternocleidomastoideus
ligamentum nuchae
ligamentum supraspinous
trapezius

BEST FOR
- sternocleidomastoideus
- trapezius
- ligamentum nuchae
- ligamentum supraspinous

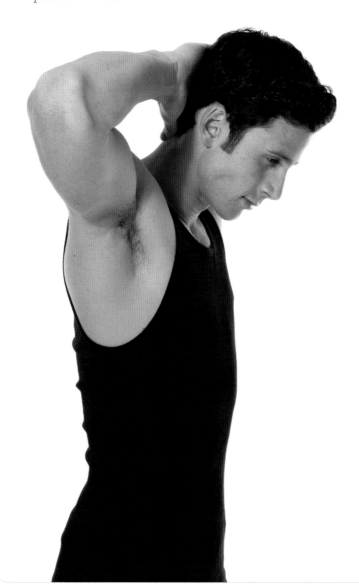

QUICK GUIDE

TARGET
- Neck

TYPE
- Flexibility

LEVEL
- Beginner

BENEFITS
- Improves range of motion
- Relieves neck pain

NOT ADVISABLE IF YOU HAVE
- Numbness running down your arm or into your hand

DO IT RIGHT

DO
- Relax your shoulder muscles.

AVOID
- Pulling too hard with your hand— this is a gentle stretch.

FLEXION ISOMETRIC

1 Sit or stand, keeping your neck, shoulders, and torso straight. Slightly flex your neck.

2 Place your palm against your forehead, and gently push your forehead into your palm, holding the position static.

3 Hold for ten seconds and release. Repeat three times.

ANNOTATION KEY
Bold text indicates active muscles
Gray text indicates stabilizing muscles
* indicates deep muscles

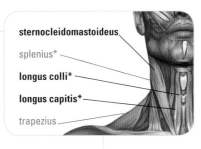

sternocleidomastoideus
splenius*
longus colli*
longus capitis*
trapezius

CERVICAL

BEST FOR
- sternocleidomastoideus
- longus colli
- longus capitis
- splenius
- trapezius

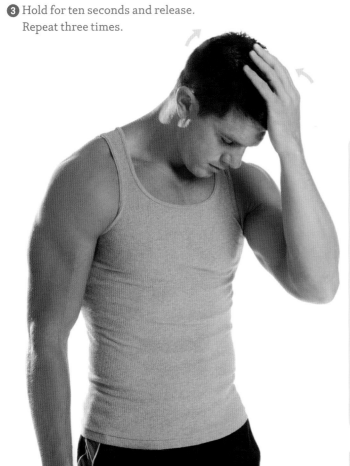

QUICK GUIDE

TARGET
- Neck flexors

TYPE
- Strengthening

LEVEL
- Beginner

BENEFITS
- Strengthens the neck flexors without irritating the ligaments, tendons, or joints

NOT ADVISABLE IF YOU HAVE
- Numbness running down your arm or into your hand

DO IT RIGHT

DO
- Apply a gentle pressure—overdoing it, especially when you first begin exercising, will make the neck muscles stiffer.

AVOID
- Any movement in the neck.

LATERAL STRETCH

CERVICAL

❶ Sit or stand, keeping your neck, shoulders, and torso straight.

❷ Tilt your head so that your right ear moves toward your right shoulder until you feel a distinct stretch in the left side of your neck.

DO IT RIGHT

DO
- Relax your shoulder muscles.

AVOID
- Rotating your head while tilting it.

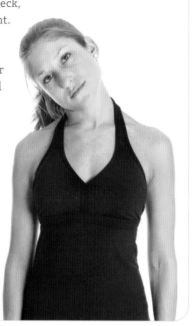

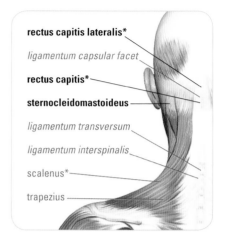

- **rectus capitis lateralis***
- *ligamentum capsular facet*
- **rectus capitis***
- **sternocleidomastoideus**
- *ligamentum transversum*
- *ligamentum interspinalis*
- scalenus*
- trapezius

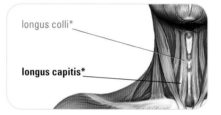

- longus colli*
- **longus capitis***

ANNOTATION KEY

Italic text indicates ligaments
Bold text indicates active muscles
Gray text indicates stabilizing muscles
* indicates deep muscles

❸ Hold for ten seconds, and repeat three times in each direction.

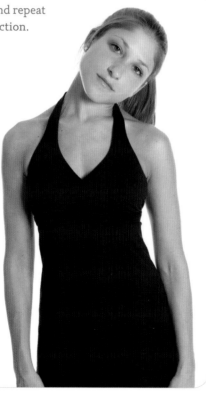

BEST FOR

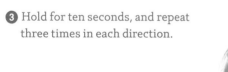

- scalenus
- sternocleidomastoideus
- trapezius
- rectus capitis lateralis
- ligamentum transversum
- ligamentum interspinalis
- ligamentum capsular facet

QUICK GUIDE

TARGET
- Neck lateral flexors

TYPE
- Flexibility

LEVEL
- Beginner

BENEFITS
- Improves range of motion
- Relieves neck pain

NOT ADVISABLE IF YOU HAVE
- Numbness running down your arm or into your hand

LATERAL ISOMETRIC

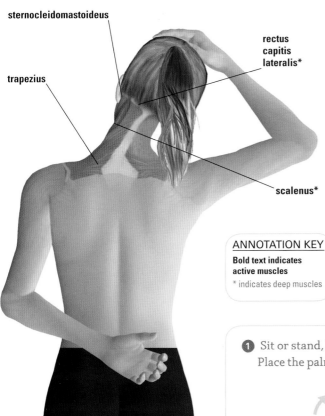

sternocleidomastoideus

trapezius

rectus
capitis
lateralis*

scalenus*

ANNOTATION KEY
Bold text indicates
active muscles
* indicates deep muscles

DO IT RIGHT

DO
• Apply a gentle pressure—
overdoing it, especially when
you first begin exercising, will
make the neck muscles stiffer.

AVOID
• Any movement in the neck.

BEST FOR

• scalenus
• sternocleidomastoideus
• trapezius
• rectus capitis lateralis

CERVICAL

QUICK GUIDE

TARGET
• Neck lateral flexors

TYPE
• Strengthening

LEVEL
• Beginner

BENEFITS
• Strengthens the lateral flexors of
the neck without irritating the
ligaments, tendons, or joints

NOT ADVISABLE IF YOU HAVE
• Numbness running down your
arm or into your hand

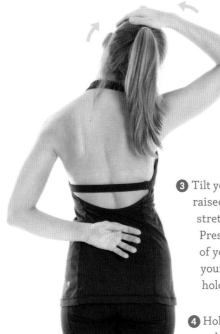

❶ Sit or stand, keeping your neck, shoulders, and torso straight.
Place the palm of your right hand on the top of your head.

❷ Reach toward the small
of your back with your
left hand, bending your
arm at the elbow.

❸ Tilt your head toward your
raised elbow until you feel the
stretch in the side of your neck.
Press your head into the palm
of your hand as you try to tilt
your ear to your shoulder,
holding the position static.

❹ Hold for ten seconds and
release. Repeat three times on
each side.

ROTATION STRETCH

CERVICAL

① Sit or stand, keeping your neck, shoulders, and torso straight. Place your right palm against your forehead.

② Turn your head slowly to the right, moving gently until you feel a stretch in the left side of your neck. Hold for ten seconds.

③ Move your head back to the forward position. Relax.

ANNOTATION KEY

Italic text indicates ligaments

Bold text indicates active muscles

Gray text indicates stabilizing muscles

* indicates deep muscles

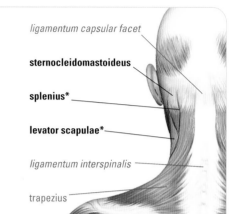

ligamentum capsular facet

sternocleidomastoideus

splenius*

levator scapulae*

ligamentum interspinalis

trapezius

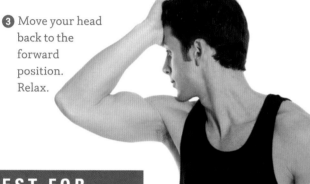

BEST FOR

- splenius
- sternocleidomastoideus
- levator scapulae
- trapezius
- ligamentum interspinalis
- ligamentum capsular facet

④ Place your left palm against your forehead, and turn your head slowly to the left, again moving gently until you feel a stretch in the right side of your neck. Hold for ten seconds.

⑤ Move your head back to the forward position. Relax, and then repeat the entire sequence five times.

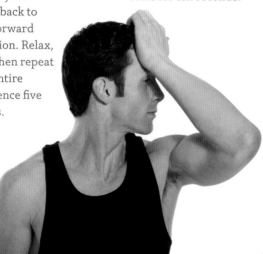

QUICK GUIDE

TARGET
- Neck rotators

TYPE
- Flexibility

LEVEL
- Beginner

BENEFITS
- Improves range of motion
- Relieves neck pain

NOT ADVISABLE IF YOU HAVE
- Numbness running down your arm or into your hand

DO IT RIGHT

DO
- Relax your shoulder muscles.
- Keep your head in a neutral position.

AVOID
- Pushing too hard with your hand—this is a gentle stretch.
- Flexing or extending your head.

ROTATION ISOMETRIC

DO IT RIGHT

DO
- Apply a gentle pressure—overdoing it, especially when you first begin exercising, will make the neck muscles stiffer.

AVOID
- Any movement in the neck.

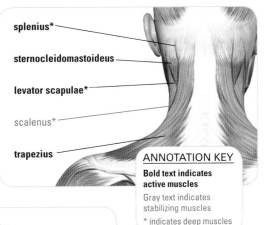

splenius*
sternocleidomastoideus
levator scapulae*
scalenus*
trapezius

ANNOTATION KEY

Bold text indicates active muscles
Gray text indicates stabilizing muscles
* indicates deep muscles

❶ Sit or stand, keeping your neck, shoulders, and torso straight. Keeping your chin level, look straight ahead.

❷ Place your left palm against your left temple, and press into your palm as if you were turning your head to the left.

❸ Hold for ten seconds and release. Repeat three times on each side.

BEST FOR
- splenius
- sternocleidomastoideus
- levator scapulae
- trapezius

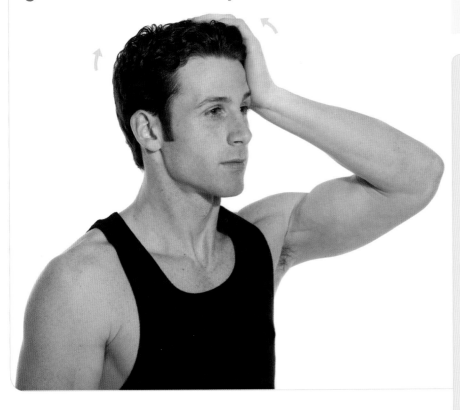

QUICK GUIDE

TARGET
- Neck rotators

TYPE
- Strengthening

LEVEL
- Beginner

BENEFITS
- Strengthens the rotary muscles of the neck without irritating the ligaments, tendons, or joints

NOT ADVISABLE IF YOU HAVE
- Numbness running down your arm or into your hand

EXTENSION STRETCH

CERVICAL

1. Sit or stand, keeping your neck, shoulders, and torso straight. Keeping your chin level, look straight ahead.

2. Gently bend your head backward so that your eyes are looking up at the ceiling. Stop when you feel a stretch in the front of your neck.

3. Hold for ten seconds, and then repeat three times.

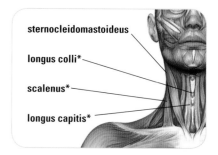

sternocleidomastoideus

longus colli*

scalenus*

longus capitis*

ANNOTATION KEY
Bold text indicates active muscles
* indicates deep muscles

BEST FOR
- scalenus
- sternocleidomastoideus
- longus colli
- longus capitis

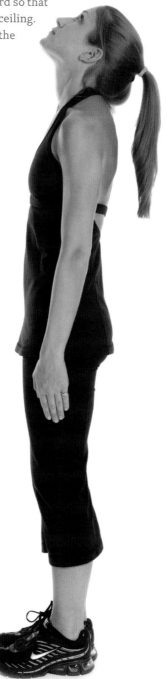

DO IT RIGHT

DO
- Relax your shoulder muscles.

AVOID
- Rotating your head while tilting it back.

QUICK GUIDE

TARGET
- Neck extensors

TYPE
- Flexibility

LEVEL
- Beginner

BENEFITS
- Improves range of motion
- Relieves neck pain

NOT ADVISABLE IF YOU HAVE
- Numbness running down your arm or into your hand

EXTENSION ISOMETRIC

CERVICAL

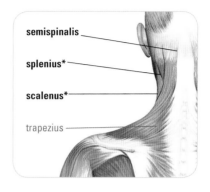

semispinalis

splenius*

scalenus*

trapezius

1. Sit or stand, keeping your neck, shoulders, and torso straight. Keeping your chin level, look straight ahead.

2. Clasp your hands together and place them behind your head.

3. Press the back of your head into your palms. Hold for ten seconds and release. Repeat three times.

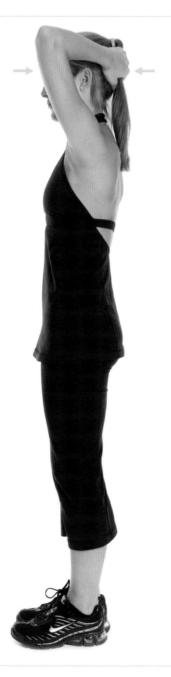

BEST FOR

- splenius
- semispinalis
- trapezius

QUICK GUIDE

TARGET
- Neck extensors

TYPE
- Strengthening

LEVEL
- Beginner

BENEFITS
- Strengthens the extensor muscles of the neck without irritating the ligaments, tendons, or joints

NOT ADVISABLE IF YOU HAVE
- Numbness running down your arm or into your hand

DO IT RIGHT

DO
- Apply a gentle pressure— overdoing it, especially when you first begin exercising, will make the neck muscles stiffer.

AVOID
- Any movement in the neck.

UPPER TRAPEZIUS STRETCH

CERVICAL

1 Sit on a Swiss ball with your feet shoulder-width apart.

2 Reach your left hand down the side of the ball, and spread your palm against the lower part of the ball.

3 With your right hand, grasp the left side of your head, and tilt your head to the right, as if you were going to touch your right ear to your right shoulder.

4 Hold for ten seconds, and return to the starting position. Repeat the entire sequence on the other side.

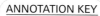

ANNOTATION KEY

Bold text indicates active muscles

Gray text indicates stabilizing muscles

* indicates deep muscles

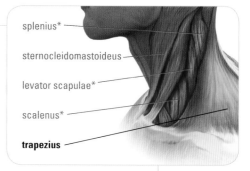

splenius*

sternocleidomastoideus

levator scapulae*

scalenus*

trapezius

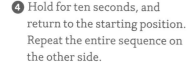

BEST FOR

• trapezius

QUICK GUIDE

TARGET
• Upper trapezius

TYPE
• Flexibility

LEVEL
• Beginner

BENEFITS
• Increases range of motion

NOT ADVISABLE IF YOU HAVE
• Neck issues

DO IT RIGHT

DO
• Grasp the side of the ball firmly to depress your shoulder blade.

AVOID
• Dropping your head forward or backward— your head should move directly to the side.

LEVATOR SCAPULAE STRETCH

1 Sit on a Swiss ball with your feet shoulder-width apart.

2 Reach your right hand down the side of the ball, and spread your palm against the lower part of the ball.

3 With your left hand, grasp the posterior right side of your head, and pull your chin in toward your lateral upper chest until you feel tension from the tip of your shoulder blade to the right side of your neck.

4 Hold for ten seconds, and return to the starting position. Repeat three times on each side.

ANNOTATION KEY
Bold text indicates active muscles
Gray text indicates stabilizing muscles
* indicates deep muscles

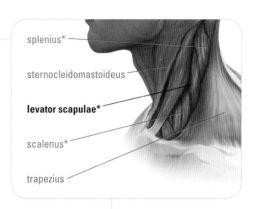

splenius*
sternocleidomastoideus
levator scapulae*
scalenus*
trapezius

CERVICAL

BEST FOR
• levator scapulae

QUICK GUIDE

TARGET
• Levator scapulae

TYPE
• Flexibility

LEVEL
• Beginner

BENEFITS
• Increases range of motion

NOT ADVISABLE IF YOU HAVE
• Neck issues

DO IT RIGHT

DO
• Grasp the side of the ball firmly to depress your shoulder blade.
• Try multiple angles to find tight muscle fibers.

AVOID
• Excessive lateral flexion.

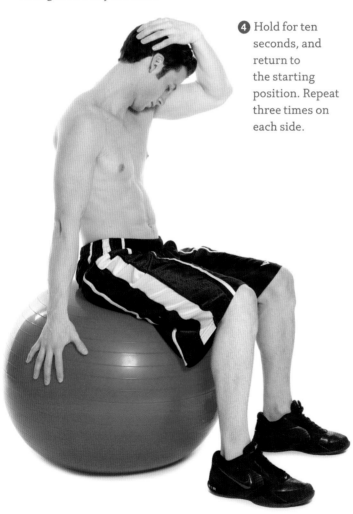

SHRUG

CERVICAL

1 Sit on a Swiss ball or chair, keeping your back straight and your head and neck centered over the rest of your spinal column.

2 With your arms at your side, bend your elbows slightly. Hold your hands with the palms up.

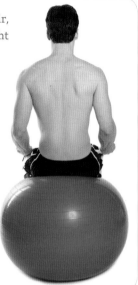

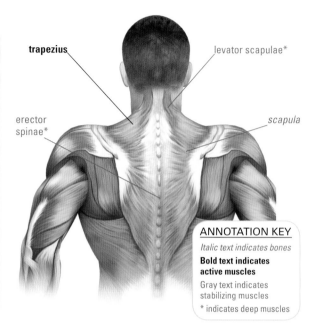

trapezius

levator scapulae*

erector spinae*

scapula

ANNOTATION KEY
Italic text indicates bones
Bold text indicates active muscles
Gray text indicates stabilizing muscles
* indicates deep muscles

DO IT RIGHT

DO
• Move in a smooth, controlled manner.

AVOID
• Rolling your shoulders—lift them directly up and down instead.

BEST FOR

• trapezius
• levator scapulae
• scapula
• erector spinae

3 Bring your shoulders down and forward, and then lift them as high as you can.

4 Repeat entire sequence five times.

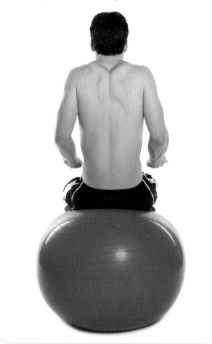

QUICK GUIDE

TARGET
• Neck
• Shoulders
• Scapula

TYPE
• Flexibility

LEVEL
• Beginner

BENEFITS
• Improves range of motion
• Relaxes tight neck, shoulder, chest, and upper-back muscles
• Stabilizes your shoulder blades

NOT ADVISABLE IF YOU HAVE
• Pain or numbness running down your arm or into your hand

TURTLE NECK

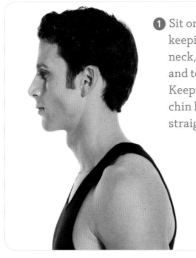

1 Sit or stand, keeping your neck, shoulders, and torso straight. Keeping your chin level, look straight ahead.

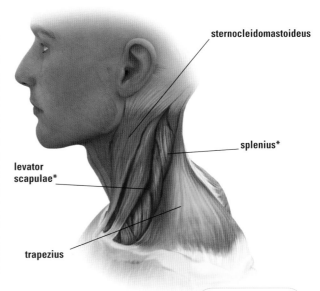

sternocleidomastoideus

splenius*

levator scapulae*

trapezius

QUICK GUIDE

TARGET
• Neck

TYPE
• Flexibility

LEVEL
• Beginner

BENEFITS
• Improves range of motion
• Corrects forward head protrusion

NOT ADVISABLE IF YOU HAVE
• Numbness running down your arm or into your hand

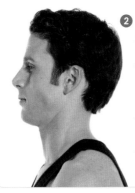

2 Move your chin in as if you were a turtle going back into its shell until you feel a stretch in the back of your neck. Hold for ten seconds.

ANNOTATION KEY
Bold text indicates active muscles
* indicates deep muscles

BEST FOR

• trapezius
• levator scapulae
• scapula
• erector spinae

DO IT RIGHT

DO
• Move in a smooth, controlled manner.

AVOID
• Lifting your chin as you move your head back.

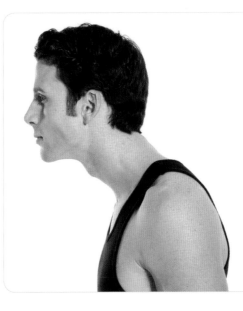

3 Extend your head forward, this time as if you were a turtle coming out of its shell. Hold for fifteen seconds.

4 Return to the starting position, and repeat five times.

CERVICAL STARS

CERVICAL

1 Sit or stand, keeping your neck, shoulders, and torso straight. Keeping your chin level, look straight ahead.

2 Imagine that there is a star in front of you with a vertical line, a horizontal line, and two diagonal lines. Trace the star shape with your head and neck by following the vertical line up and down three times.

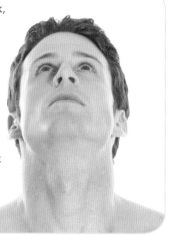

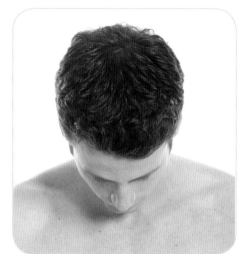

3 Next, follow the horizontal line once.

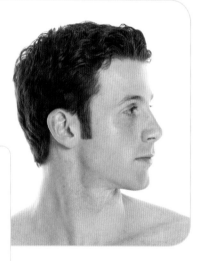

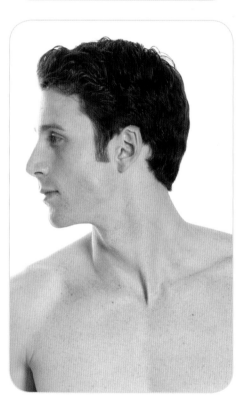

QUICK GUIDE

TARGET
- Neck rotators
- Neck flexors
- Neck extensors
- Neck lateral flexors

TYPE
- Flexibility

LEVEL
- Beginner

BENEFITS
- Improves range of motion
- Relieves neck pain

NOT ADVISABLE IF YOU HAVE
- Numbness running down your arm or into your hand

BEST FOR
- splenius
- sternocleidomastoideus
- levator scapulae
- scalenus
- semispinalis
- trapezius

4 Finally, trace the two diagonal lines.

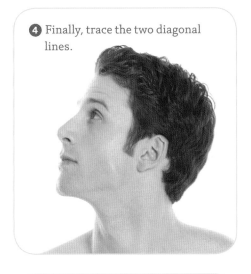

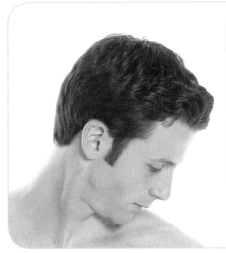

DO IT RIGHT

DO
• Move in a smooth, controlled manner.

AVOID
• Hunching or tensing your shoulders.

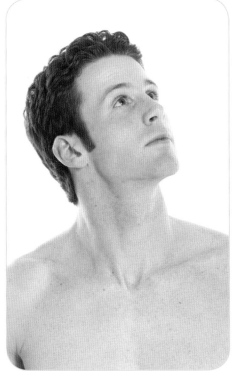

5 Return to the start position, and repeat five times.

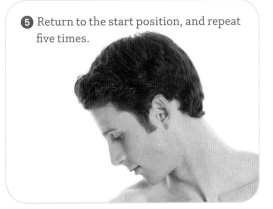

ANNOTATION KEY
Bold text indicates active muscles
* indicates deep muscles

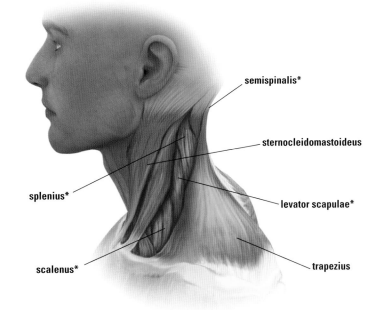

semispinalis*

sternocleidomastoideus

splenius*

levator scapulae*

scalenus*

trapezius

THORACIC EXERCISES

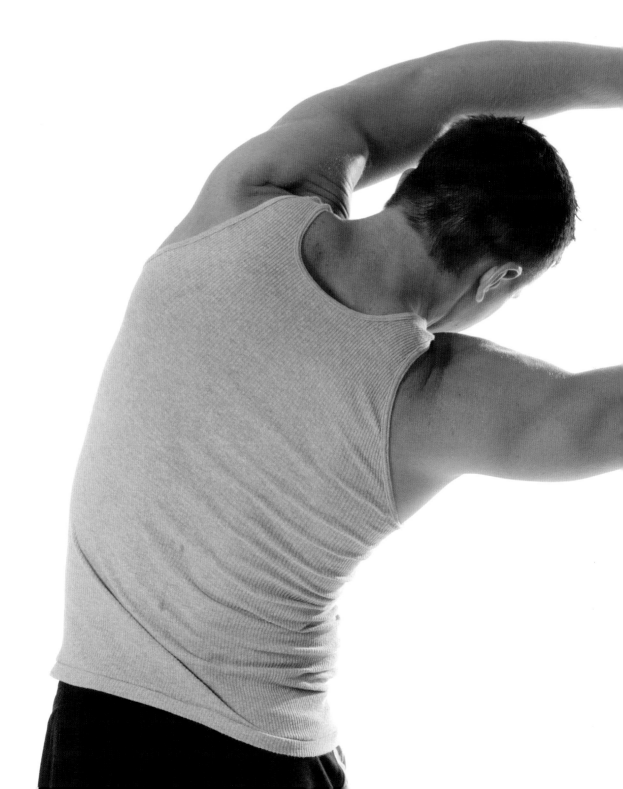

As with many back complaints, pain in the upper, or thoracic, is often the result of poor posture. So many of us spend long days—and nights—sitting bent forward over a computer keyboard, whether working or "relaxing." Upper-back pain is also prevalent in those who do a lot of lifting, from retail workers stocking store shelves to mothers toting infants. Athletes, from pro pitchers lobbing a fastball to "weekend warriors" tossing a football, are also prone to thoracic and shoulder pain. As well as pain between the shoulder blades, thoracic issues, whether a result of poor posture, heavy lifting, or injury, can produce symptoms such as difficulty in taking deep breaths or even pain in the front of the chest.

Working on improving your posture and lifting habits and making sure that you sit in a good chair with a firm back support can help relieve thoracic spine stiffness or pain. And to further promote a healthy back, add exercises that target your thoracic spine, shoulders, and chest.

SCAPULAR RANGE OF MOTION

THORACIC

1 Sit or stand, keeping your neck, shoulders, and torso in a relaxed, neutral position. Keeping your chin level, look straight ahead.

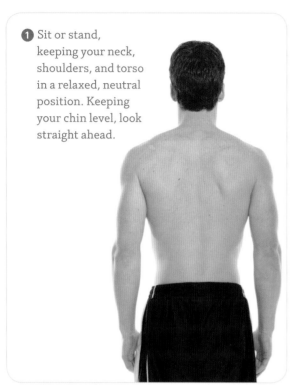

2 With your arms at your side, bend your elbows slightly. Hold your hands with the palms up.

3 Roll your shoulders forward, concentrating on separating your scapula from your spine.

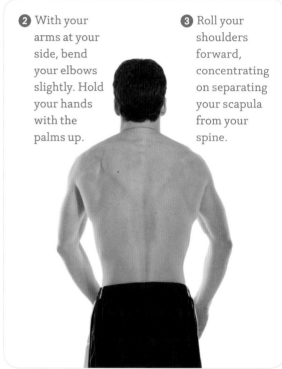

4 Roll your shoulders back and slightly upward, squeezing your scapulae together.

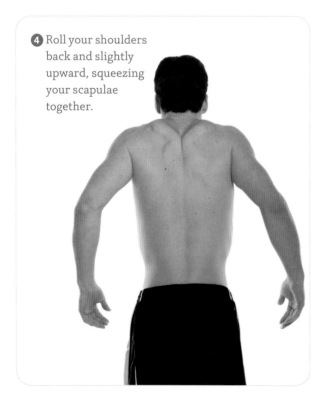

5 Roll your shoulders down and backward.

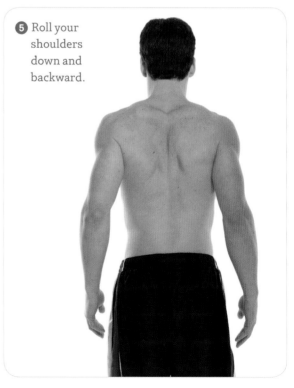

DO IT RIGHT

DO
• Move your shoulders in a smooth, controlled manner.

AVOID
• Moving your torso.

ANNOTATION KEY

Italic text indicates bones
Bold text indicates active muscles
Gray text indicates stabilizing muscles
* indicates deep muscles

BEST FOR

• trapezius
• levator scapulae
• scapula
• erector spinae

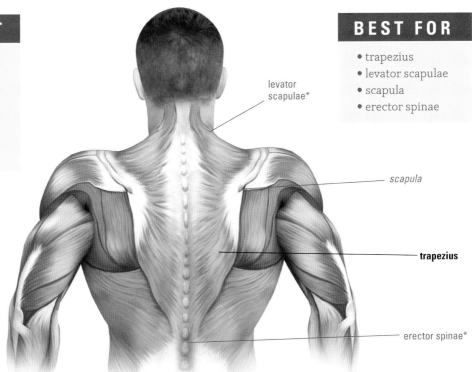

levator scapulae*

scapula

trapezius

erector spinae*

6 Lower your shoulders while continuing to squeeze your scapulae together.

7 Lower your shoulders to the neutral starting position.

8 Repeat entire sequence three times.

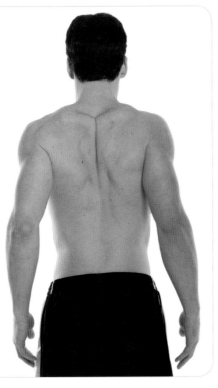

QUICK GUIDE

TARGET
• Shoulders
• Scapula
• Neck

TYPE
• Flexibility

LEVEL
• Beginner

BENEFITS
• Improves range of motion
• Relaxes tight neck, shoulder, chest, and upper-back muscles
• Stabilizes your shoulder blades

NOT ADVISABLE IF YOU HAVE
• Shoulder injury

SHOULDER STRETCH I

THORACIC

1 Sit or stand, keeping your neck, shoulders, and torso straight.

2 Raise your right arm, and bend it behind your head.

3 Keeping your shoulders relaxed, grasp your raised elbow with your left hand, and gently pull back.

4 Continue to pull your elbow back until you feel the stretch on the underside of your arm. Hold for fifteen seconds.

5 Repeat three times on each arm.

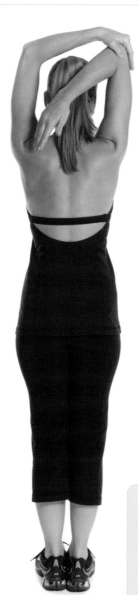

BEST FOR

- triceps brachii
- infraspinatus
- teres major
- teres minor
- latissimus dorsi

ANNOTATION KEY

Bold text indicates active muscles

Gray text indicates stabilizing muscles

* indicates deep muscles

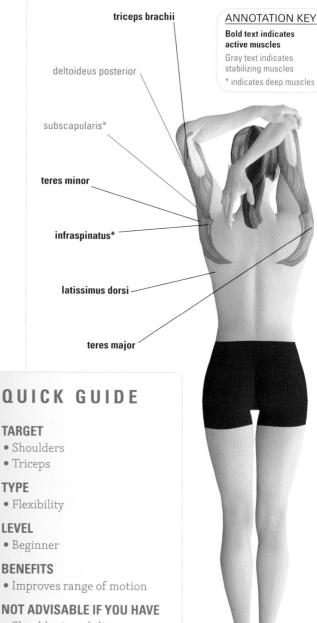

triceps brachii

deltoideus posterior

subscapularis*

teres minor

infraspinatus*

latissimus dorsi

teres major

QUICK GUIDE

TARGET
- Shoulders
- Triceps

TYPE
- Flexibility

LEVEL
- Beginner

BENEFITS
- Improves range of motion

NOT ADVISABLE IF YOU HAVE
- Shoulder instability

DO IT RIGHT

DO
- Keep your dropped elbow close to the side of your head.

AVOID
- Leaning backward.

SHOULDER STRETCH II

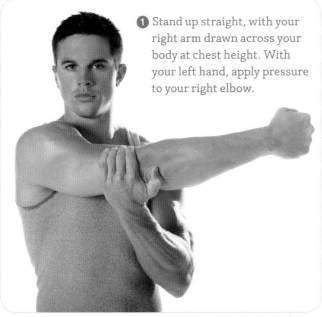

1 Stand up straight, with your right arm drawn across your body at chest height. With your left hand, apply pressure to your right elbow.

BEST FOR

- deltoideus posterior
- triceps brachii
- teres minor
- obliquus externus
- infraspinatus

2 Hold for fifteen seconds, release, and repeat three times. Repeat three times on left arm.

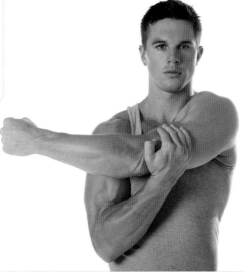

THORACIC

DO IT RIGHT

DO
- Keep your elbow straight while you apply pressure with your hand.

AVOID
- Lifting your shoulders toward your ears.

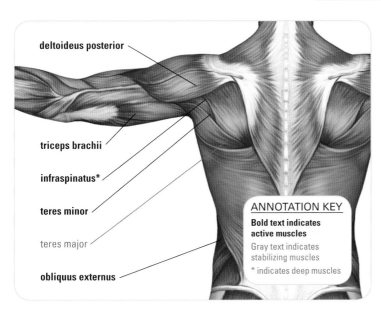

deltoideus posterior

triceps brachii

infraspinatus*

teres minor

teres major

obliquus externus

ANNOTATION KEY
Bold text indicates active muscles
Gray text indicates stabilizing muscles
* indicates deep muscles

QUICK GUIDE

TARGET
- Shoulders

TYPE
- Stretching/flexibility

LEVEL
- Beginner

BENEFITS
- Stretches posterior deltoid

NOT ADVISABLE IF YOU HAVE
- Rotator cuff injury
- Shoulder instability

SIDE BENDING

THORACIC

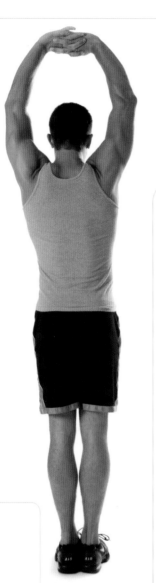

❶ Stand, keeping your neck, shoulders, and torso straight.

❷ Raise both arms above your head and clasp your hands together, palms facing upward.

DO IT RIGHT

DO
• Elongate your arms and shoulders as much as possible.

AVOID
• Dropping to the side too quickly.

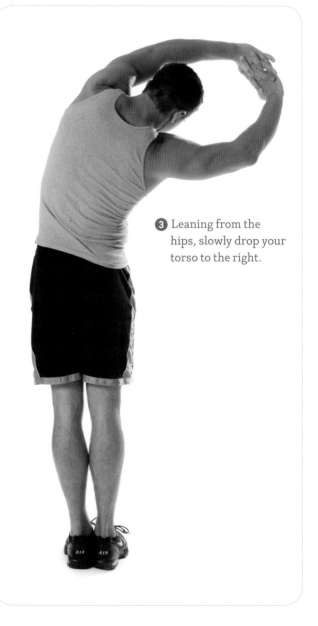

❸ Leaning from the hips, slowly drop your torso to the right.

QUICK GUIDE

TARGET
• Upper back
• Obliques

TYPE
• Flexibility

LEVEL
• Beginner

BENEFITS
• Helps correct bad posture

NOT ADVISABLE IF YOU HAVE
• Lower-back pain

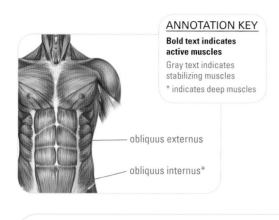

ANNOTATION KEY

Bold text indicates active muscles
Gray text indicates stabilizing muscles
* indicates deep muscles

obliquus externus

obliquus internus*

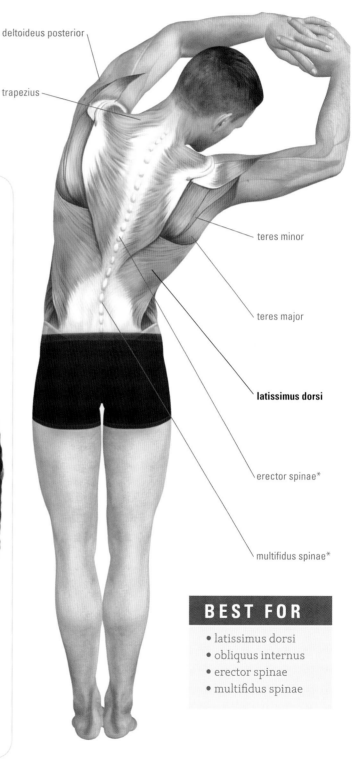

deltoideus posterior

trapezius

teres minor

teres major

latissimus dorsi

erector spinae*

multifidus spinae*

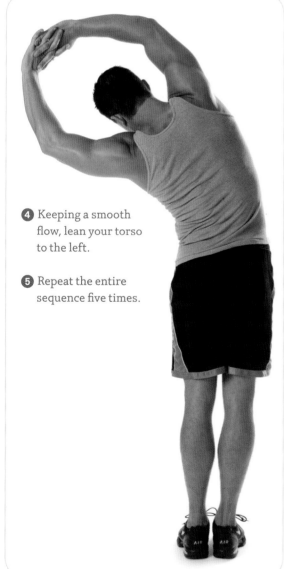

④ Keeping a smooth flow, lean your torso to the left.

⑤ Repeat the entire sequence five times.

BEST FOR

- latissimus dorsi
- obliquus internus
- erector spinae
- multifidus spinae

LATISSIMUS DORSI STRETCH

THORACIC

① Stand, keeping your neck, shoulders, and torso straight.

② Raise both arms above your head and clasp your hands together, palms facing upward.

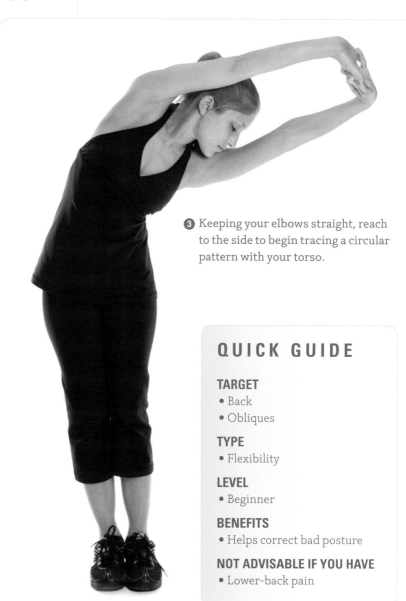

DO IT RIGHT

DO
• Elongate your arms and shoulders as much as possible.

AVOID
• Leaning backward as you come to the top of the circle.

③ Keeping your elbows straight, reach to the side to begin tracing a circular pattern with your torso.

QUICK GUIDE

TARGET
• Back
• Obliques

TYPE
• Flexibility

LEVEL
• Beginner

BENEFITS
• Helps correct bad posture

NOT ADVISABLE IF YOU HAVE
• Lower-back pain

4 Lean forward and then to the opposite side as you slowly trace a full circle.

5 Return to the starting position, and then repeat the sequence three times in each direction.

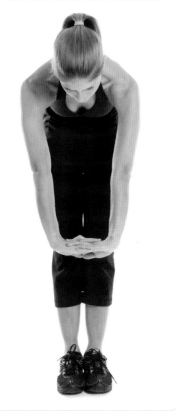

BEST FOR

- latissimus dorsi
- obliquus internus

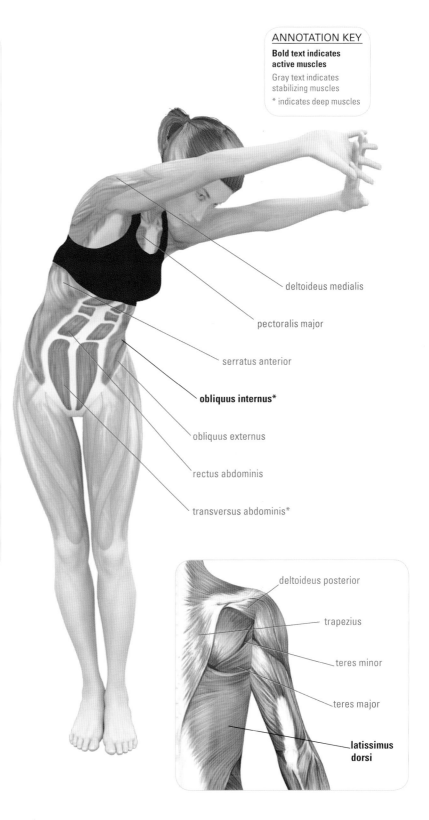

ANNOTATION KEY

Bold text indicates active muscles
Gray text indicates stabilizing muscles
* indicates deep muscles

deltoideus medialis

pectoralis major

serratus anterior

obliquus internus*

obliquus externus

rectus abdominis

transversus abdominis*

deltoideus posterior

trapezius

teres minor

teres major

latissimus dorsi

PECTORAL STRETCH

THORACIC

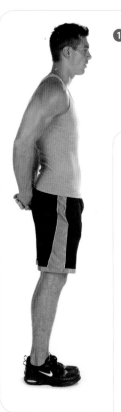

1 Stand straight with your arms behind your back and your hands clasped together.

ANNOTATION KEY

Bold text indicates active muscles
Gray text indicates stabilizing muscles
* indicates deep muscles

2 Pinch your shoulder blades together as you reach and lift your arms away from your body, making sure to keep your elbows straight.

3 Hold for fifteen seconds before returning your arms to the starting position. Repeat three times.

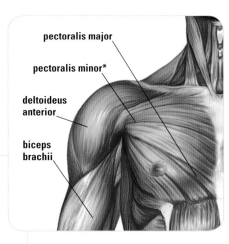

pectoralis major
pectoralis minor*
deltoideus anterior
biceps brachii

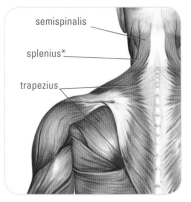

semispinalis
splenius*
trapezius

QUICK GUIDE

TARGET
• Upper back
• Chest

TYPE
• Flexibility

LEVEL
• Beginner

BENEFITS
• Stabilizes core
• Stretches chest muscles

NOT ADVISABLE IF YOU HAVE
• Neck issues
• Lower-back pain

BEST FOR

• pectoralis major
• pectoralis minor
• deltoideus anterior
• biceps brachii

DO IT RIGHT

DO
• Keep your elbows straight during the movement.

AVOID
• Leaning your trunk too far forward while stretching—this can be harmful to your back.

OPEN BOOK STRETCH

THORACIC

① Lie on your side, and cross your right leg over your left with your right knee bent.

② Place your left hand on your right knee to keep your knee from moving. With your right hand, grab your rib cage.

ANNOTATION KEY
Bold text indicates active muscles
* indicates deep muscles

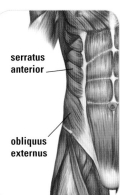

serratus anterior

obliquus externus

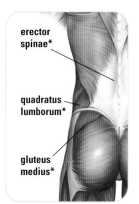

erector spinae*

quadratus lumborum*

gluteus medius*

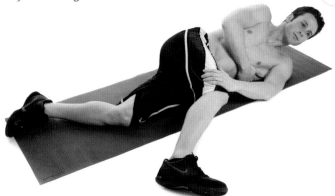

BEST FOR

- quadratus lumborum
- erector spinae
- obliquus externus
- gluteus medius
- serratus anterior

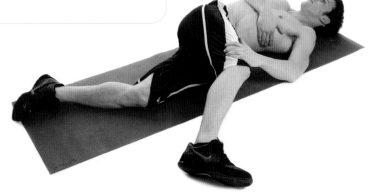

QUICK GUIDE

TARGET
- Middle back
- Chest
- Gluteal muscles

TYPE
- Flexibility

LEVEL
- Beginner

BENEFITS
- Increases thoracic flexibility
- Opens up rib cage

NOT ADVISABLE IF YOU HAVE
- Severe lower-back pain

③ Rotate your trunk to the right, stretching as far as possible. Hold for fifteen seconds.

④ Repeat the stretch, moving to the left side.

DO IT RIGHT

DO
- Keep your lower leg flat on the floor.
- Touch both shoulders to the floor.

AVOID
- Bouncing while stretching—move slowly and smoothly.

CHAIR TWIST

THORACIC

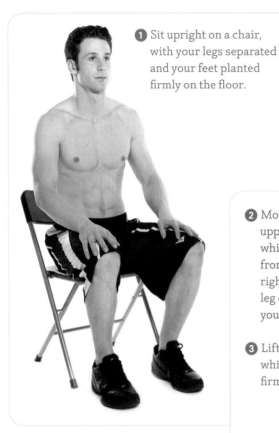

① Sit upright on a chair, with your legs separated and your feet planted firmly on the floor.

DO IT RIGHT

DO
• Move carefully—lower yourself to only as far as you feel a distinct stretch. As you become more flexible, you can deepen the stretch.

AVOID
• Lifting your buttocks off the chair.

② Moving slowly, extend your upper back and lean forward while twisting to the left from the waist. Reach your right hand to the front left leg of the chair to stabilize your body.

④ Slowly return to the starting position, and then reach to the right side. Repeat five times in each direction.

③ Lift and rotate your torso while keeping your hand firmly on the chair leg.

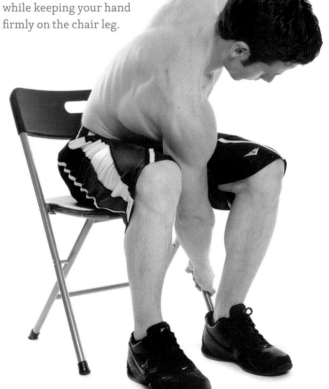

QUICK GUIDE

TARGET
• Upper back
• Back extensors
• Obliques

TYPE
• Flexibility

LEVEL
• Beginner

BENEFITS
• Increases thoracic rotation
• Stretches rhomboid muscles

NOT ADVISABLE IF YOU HAVE
• Torn rotator cuff
• Shoulder instability

BEST FOR

- iliocostalis thoracis
- multifidus spinae
- obliquus externus
- obliquus internus

obliquus externus

obliquus internus*

longissimus thoracis

erector spinae*

multifidus spinae*

latissimus dorsi

quadratus
lumborum*

**iliocostalis
thoracis***

rhomboideus*

deltoideus posterior

ANNOTATION KEY

Bold text indicates active muscles

Gray text indicates
stabilizing muscles

* indicates deep muscles

POSTERIOR HAND CLASP

THORACIC

1 Sit or stand, keeping your neck, shoulders, and torso straight. Your arms should hang loosely at your sides.

2 Extend your right hand to the side, parallel to the floor.

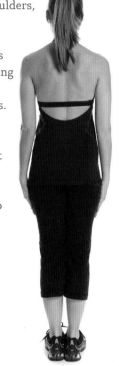

3 Bend your elbow, and rotate your shoulder downward so that the palm of your hand faces behind you. Reach behind your back, palm still up, and draw your elbow into your right side.

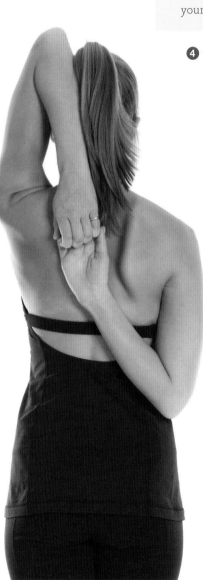

4 Continue to rotate your shoulder downward as you reach upward with your hand until your forearm is parallel to your spine. Your right hand should rest in between your shoulder blades.

5 Reach your left arm up with your palm facing directly behind you. Bend your elbow, reaching your left hand down the center of your back.

6 Hook your hands together behind your back. Lift your chest, and pull your abdominals in toward your spine.

7 Hold for about thirty seconds to one minute. Release your arms, and repeat with your arms reversed for the same length of time.

QUICK GUIDE

TARGET
• Upper back
• Upper arms

TYPE
• Flexibility

LEVEL
• Intermediate

BENEFITS
• Stretches the shoulders, chest, and upper arms

NOT ADVISABLE IF YOU HAVE
• Shoulder injury

BEST FOR

- rhomboideus
- teres minor
- subscapularis
- latissimus dorsi
- deltoideus anterior
- deltoideus medialis
- deltoideus posterior
- triceps brachii
- pectoralis major
- pectoralis minor

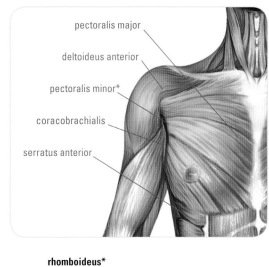

pectoralis major

deltoideus anterior

pectoralis minor*

coracobrachialis

serratus anterior

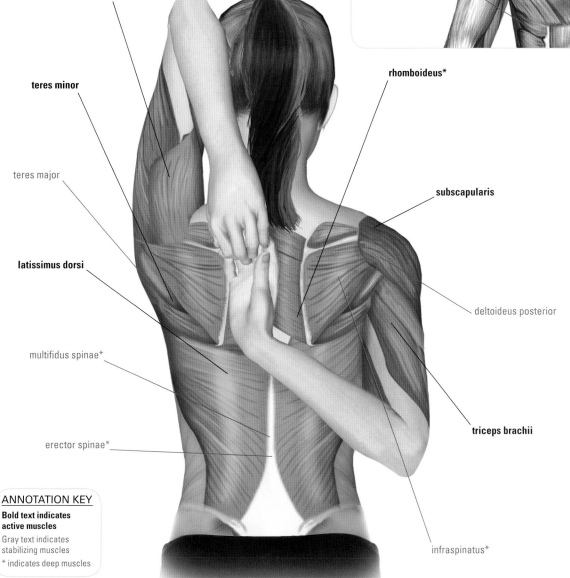

deltoideus medialis

teres minor

teres major

latissimus dorsi

multifidus spinae*

erector spinae*

rhomboideus*

subscapularis

deltoideus posterior

triceps brachii

infraspinatus*

ANNOTATION KEY

Bold text indicates active muscles

Gray text indicates stabilizing muscles

* indicates deep muscles

HAND WALKOUT

THORACIC

1 Lie prone on a Swiss ball, with your hips over the center of the ball as you support your weight on your arms. Your hands should be directly below your shoulders.

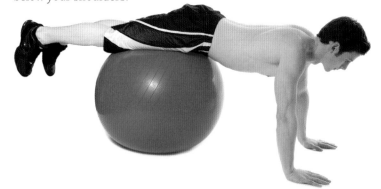

2 Lift, reach, and place your left hand forward, rolling the ball underneath you until it reaches your feet.

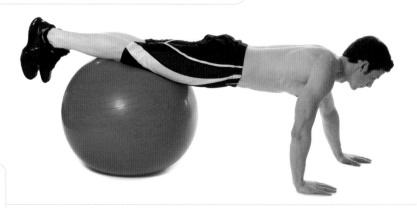

QUICK GUIDE

TARGET
- Shoulders
- Upper back
- Core muscles

TYPE
- Strengthening/stability

LEVEL
- Intermediate

BENEFITS
- Strengthens shoulders
- Stabilizes core
- Strengthens abdominals

NOT ADVISABLE IF YOU HAVE
- Wrist pain
- Lower-back pain
- Shoulder instability

3 Hold for five seconds, and then walk your hands backward, rolling the ball back underneath you until you reach the starting position.

4 Repeat the entire sequence five times.

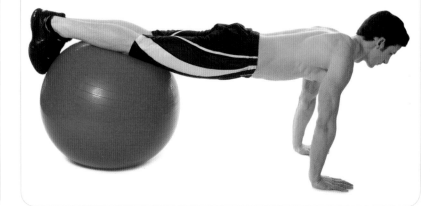

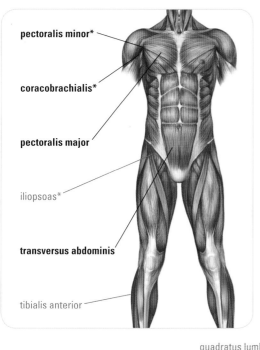

pectoralis minor*

coracobrachialis*

pectoralis major

iliopsoas*

transversus abdominis

tibialis anterior

DO IT RIGHT

DO
• Form a straight plane from neck to ankles.
• Activate your abdominals as you straighten your back.

AVOID
• Arching your back during the exercise.
• Allowing your hips to rotate.
• Locking your elbows.
• Reaching too far forward—start with a short position reach and progressively increase the length as you gain stability.

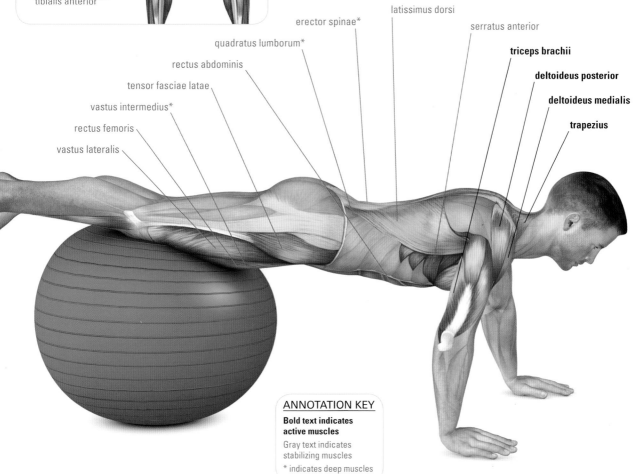

latissimus dorsi

erector spinae*

quadratus lumborum*

serratus anterior

triceps brachii

rectus abdominis

deltoideus posterior

tensor fasciae latae

deltoideus medialis

vastus intermedius*

trapezius

rectus femoris

vastus lateralis

ANNOTATION KEY
Bold text indicates active muscles
Gray text indicates stabilizing muscles
* indicates deep muscles

HAND WALK-AROUND

THORACIC

❶ Lie prone on a Swiss ball, and move forward until just your shins and upper feet are propped on the ball as you support your weight on your arms. Your hands should be directly below your shoulders.

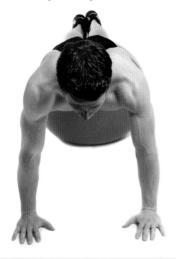

BEST FOR

- deltoideus anterior
- deltoideus medialis
- deltoideus posterior
- triceps brachii
- transversus abdominis
- pectoralis major
- pectoralis minor

❷ Lift, reach, and place your left hand to the side, followed by the right hand, as you "walk" in a circle.

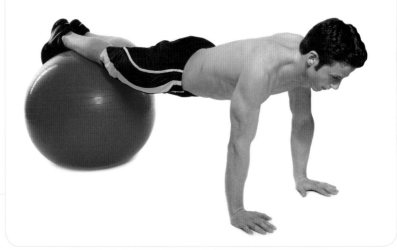

QUICK GUIDE

TARGET
- Shoulders
- Upper back
- Core muscles

TYPE
- Strengthening/stability

LEVEL
- Intermediate

BENEFITS
- Strengthens shoulders
- Stabilizes core
- Strengthens abdominals

NOT ADVISABLE IF YOU HAVE
- Wrist pain
- Lower-back pain
- Shoulder instability

❸ Rotate 90 degrees to your left, or a quarter turn, and then hand walk back to the starting position.

❹ Repeat the entire sequence, moving to the right.

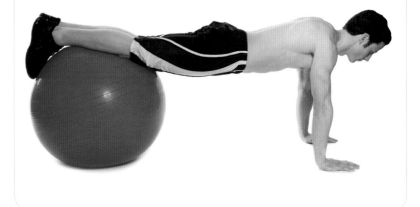

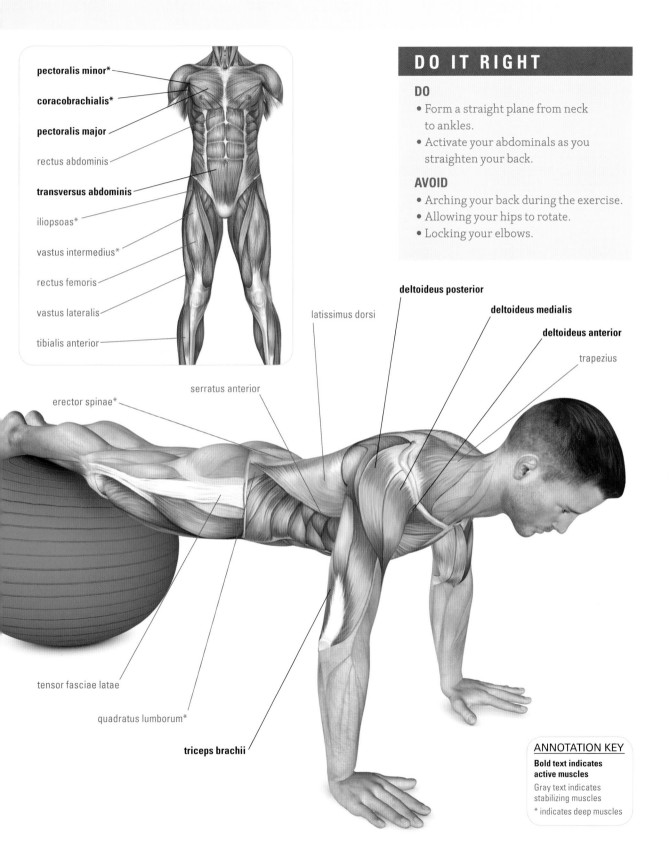

pectoralis minor*

coracobrachialis*

pectoralis major

rectus abdominis

transversus abdominis

iliopsoas*

vastus intermedius*

rectus femoris

vastus lateralis

tibialis anterior

DO IT RIGHT

DO
- Form a straight plane from neck to ankles.
- Activate your abdominals as you straighten your back.

AVOID
- Arching your back during the exercise.
- Allowing your hips to rotate.
- Locking your elbows.

deltoideus posterior

deltoideus medialis

deltoideus anterior

trapezius

latissimus dorsi

serratus anterior

erector spinae*

tensor fasciae latae

quadratus lumborum*

triceps brachii

ANNOTATION KEY

Bold text indicates active muscles

Gray text indicates stabilizing muscles

* indicates deep muscles

SWISS BALL REVERSE FLY

THORACIC

❶ Lie prone on the Swiss ball, with your legs stretched out and toes on the floor. Take hold of small hand weights with a palms-in, neutral grip. Start with your arms extended downward with a slight bend in the elbows.

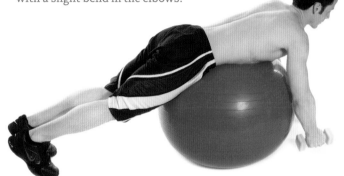

DO IT RIGHT

DO
• Keep a slight bend in your elbows throughout the entire exercise.
• Raise your elbows as high as you can, so that they both reach the same height.

AVOID
• Moving your torso during the exercise.
• Allowing the weights to touch the floor.

❷ Lift your elbows just past shoulder level, keeping your arms in a fixed position.

❸ Hold for five seconds, and then lower your arms, returning the weights almost to the floor. Repeat ten times.

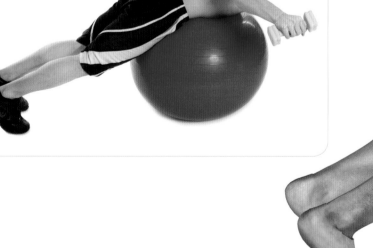

QUICK GUIDE

TARGET
• Back
• Chest

TYPE
• Strengthening/stretching

LEVEL
• Intermediate

BENEFITS
• Strengthens upper back and shoulders
• Stretches chest muscles

NOT ADVISABLE IF YOU HAVE
• Neck issues
• Lower-back pain

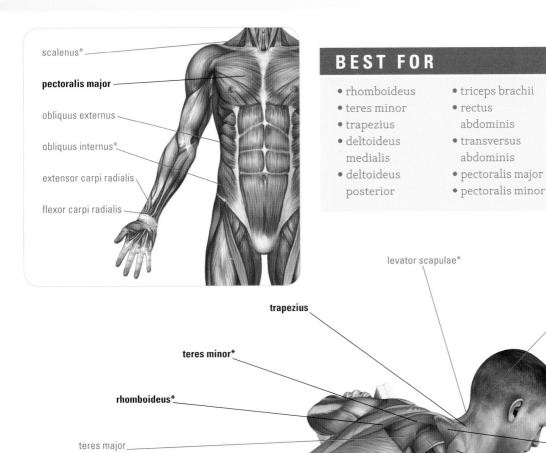

scalenus*

pectoralis major

obliquus externus

obliquus internus*

extensor carpi radialis

flexor carpi radialis

BEST FOR

- rhomboideus
- teres minor
- trapezius
- deltoideus medialis
- deltoideus posterior
- triceps brachii
- rectus abdominis
- transversus abdominis
- pectoralis major
- pectoralis minor

levator scapulae*

splenius*

trapezius

teres minor*

rhomboideus*

teres major

latissimus dorsi

quadratus lumborum*

deltoideus posterior

deltoideus medialis

brachioradialis

triceps brachii

ANNOTATION KEY

Bold text indicates active muscles

Gray text indicates stabilizing muscles

* indicates deep muscles

SWISS BALL ROW

THORACIC

1 Place two small hand weights on the side of a Swiss ball. Lie facedown on the ball with your legs stretched out straight behind you and your toes on the floor.

2 Grasp each weight with an overhand grip, with your arms extended down toward the floor, your hands pronated. This is your starting position.

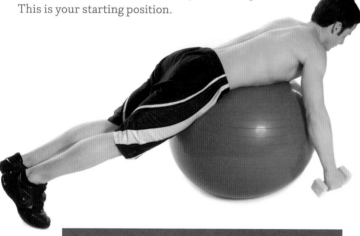

QUICK GUIDE

TARGET
• Upper back
• Shoulders
• Upper arms

TYPE
• Strengthening

LEVEL
• Intermediate

BENEFITS
• Strengthens upper back and shoulders
• Tones upper arms

NOT ADVISABLE IF YOU HAVE
• Severe neck pain
• Severe lower-back pain
• Shoulder instability

BEST FOR

• trapezius
• rhomboideus
• rectus femoris
• deltoideus posterior
• biceps brachii
• latissimus dorsi
• teres major
• teres minor

3 Lift your elbows up past shoulder level, bending your arms at a 90-degree angle.

4 Pause, squeeze your shoulder blades together, and then extend your arms, returning the weights back toward the floor.

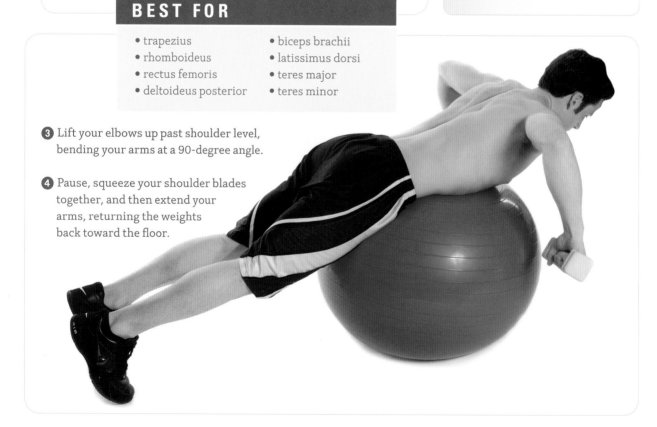

DO IT RIGHT

DO
- Keep your forearms vertical throughout the exercise.
- Exhale as you flex your arms and lift your elbows, and inhale as you extend your arms down.
- Keep your legs straight.

AVOID
- Allowing the weights to touch the floor.
- Moving your torso.

sternocleimastoideus

scalenus*

pectoralis major

biceps brachii

ANNOTATION KEY
Bold text indicates active muscles
Gray text indicates stabilizing muscles
* indicates deep muscles

deltoideus posterior

trapezius

levator scapulae*

splenius*

infraspinatus*

triceps brachii

teres minor

rhomboideus*

subscapularis*

teres major

latissimus dorsi

erector spinae*

brachialis

quadratus lumborum*

gluteus maximus

vastus lateralis

vastus intermedius*

tibialis anterior

rectus femoris

tibialis posterior*

soleus

vastus medialis*

peroneus

extensor hallucis

flexor hallucis*

extensor digitorum

BODY BALL EXTENSION

THORACIC

❶ Lie supine over a Swiss ball, with your upper chest and head hanging off the edge of the ball.

DO IT RIGHT

DO
- Keep your glutes and thighs constantly engaged while you perform this exercise.
- Keep your lower body taut.
- Keep your head in neutral position.
- Keep a wide base for extra balance.

AVOID
- Elevating your shoulders.
- Lifting your hip bones off the ball.

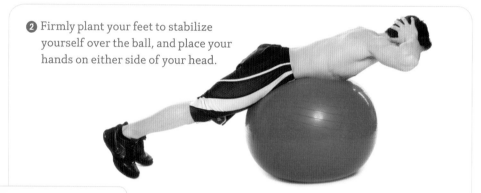

❷ Firmly plant your feet to stabilize yourself over the ball, and place your hands on either side of your head.

QUICK GUIDE

TARGET
- Middle back
- Lower back

TYPE
- Strengthening/stability

LEVEL
- Advanced

BENEFITS
- Stabilizes core
- Strengthens back extensor muscles
- Strengthens abdominals

NOT ADVISABLE IF YOU HAVE
- Neck issues
- Lower-back pain

❸ With arms bent and elbows out, raise your upper body about eight to twelve inches off the ball.

❹ Slowly and carefully lower your body to the starting position. Repeat ten times.

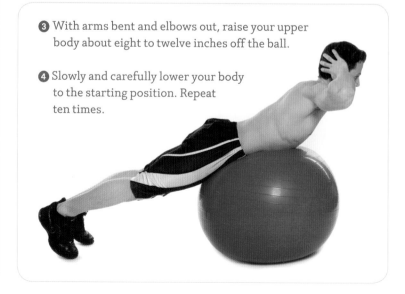

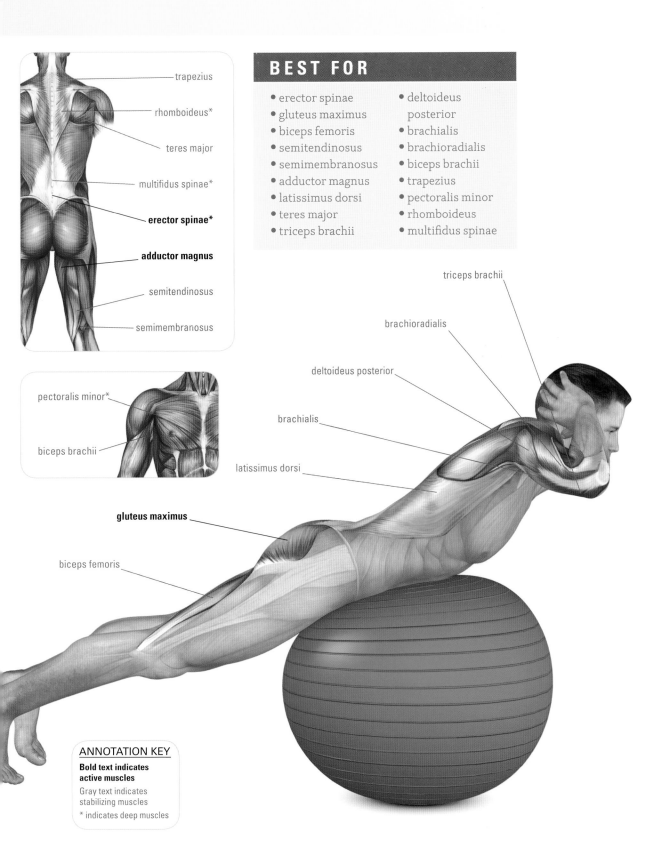

BEST FOR

- erector spinae
- gluteus maximus
- biceps femoris
- semitendinosus
- semimembranosus
- adductor magnus
- latissimus dorsi
- teres major
- triceps brachii
- deltoideus posterior
- brachialis
- brachioradialis
- biceps brachii
- trapezius
- pectoralis minor
- rhomboideus
- multifidus spinae

trapezius

rhomboideus*

teres major

multifidus spinae*

erector spinae*

adductor magnus

semitendinosus

semimembranosus

pectoralis minor*

biceps brachii

gluteus maximus

biceps femoris

triceps brachii

brachioradialis

deltoideus posterior

brachialis

latissimus dorsi

ANNOTATION KEY

Bold text indicates active muscles

Gray text indicates stabilizing muscles

* indicates deep muscles

BACKWARD BALL STRETCH

THORACIC

1 Sit on a Swiss ball in a well-balanced, neutral position, with your hips directly over the center of the ball.

2 Raise your arms while maintaining good balance, and begin to extend them behind you.

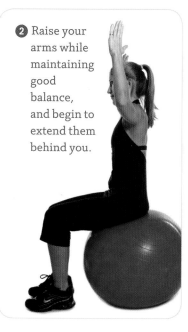

DO IT RIGHT

DO
- Maintain good balance throughout the stretch.
- Move slowly and in a controlled manner.
- Keep your head on the ball until you have dropped your knees all the way down as you release from the stretch.

AVOID
- Lateral ball movement.
- Holding the extended position for too long, or until you feel dizzy.

3 As you continue to extend your hands backward, walk your feet forward, allowing the ball to roll up your spine.

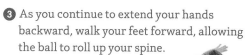

4 As your hands touch the floor, extend your legs as far forward as you comfortably can. Hold this position for ten seconds.

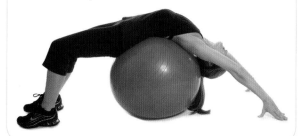

5 To deepen the stretch, extend your arms, and walk your legs and hands closer to the ball. Hold this position for ten seconds.

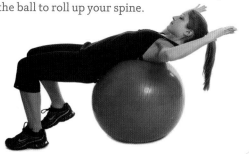
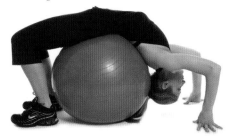

6 To release the stretch, bend your knees, drop your hips to the floor, lift your head off the ball, and then walk back to the starting position.

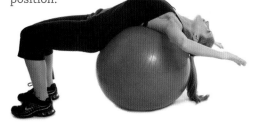

QUICK GUIDE

TARGET
- Thoracic and upper lumbar spine
- Abdominals

TYPE
- Flexibility

LEVEL
- Advanced

BENEFITS
- Stretches thoracic spine
- Increases spinal extension
- Stretches abdominals and latissimus dorsi muscles

NOT ADVISABLE IF YOU HAVE
- Lower-back pain
- Balancing difficulty
- Vestibular deficits

MODIFICATION
Easier: Follow steps 1 through 3, but rather than extend your hands to the floor, clasp them behind your head. Hold this position for ten seconds, and release.

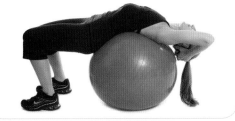

BEST FOR
- deltoideus medialis
- iliopsoas
- latissimus dorsi
- serratus anterior
- pectoralis major
- pectoralis minor
- ligamentum longitudinale anterius

ANNOTATION KEY
Italic text indicates ligaments
Bold text indicates active muscles
Gray text indicates stabilizing muscles
* indicates deep muscles

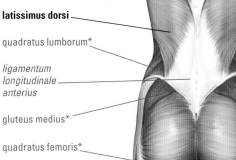

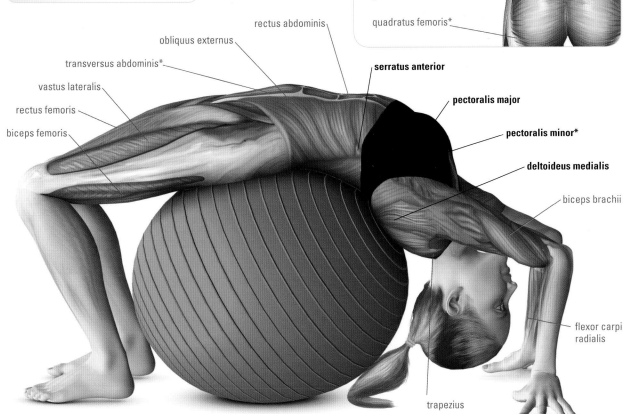

CORE EXERCISES

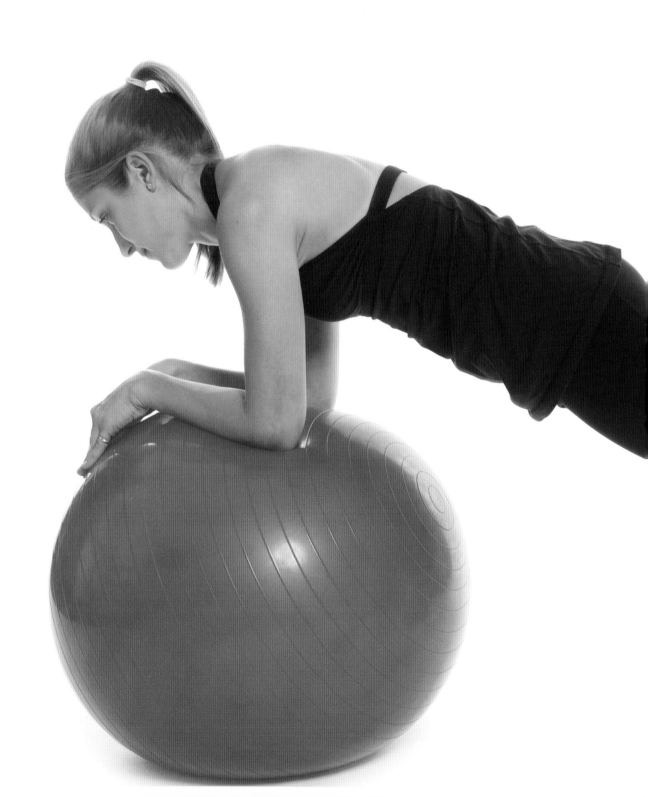

What are the core muscles—and why are they so crucial to a healthy back? The major core muscles are the deep muscle layers that lie close to the spine, including the abdominals (the rectus abdominis, transversus abdominis, obliquus externus, and obliquus internus), the pelvic floor muscles (the levator ani, pubococcygeus, iliococcygeus, puborectalis, and coccygeus), the spinal extensors (multifidus spinae, erector spinae, splenius, longissimus thoracis, and semispinalis), and the diaphragm. These muscles provide structural support for the entire body. The minor core muscles include the latissimus dorsi, gluteus maximus, and trapezius. Together, the core muscles are responsible for nearly all of your everyday movements, and they stabilize your trunk and pelvis, allowing your arms and legs to move properly. Exercising these important muscles to stabilize, strengthen, and align the body is crucial to a healthy back. A strong core makes it easier to move with any activity. Well-conditioned core muscles also allow you to maintain good posture. Deconditioned or weak core muscles leave you predisposed to injury.

SITTING BALANCE

CORE

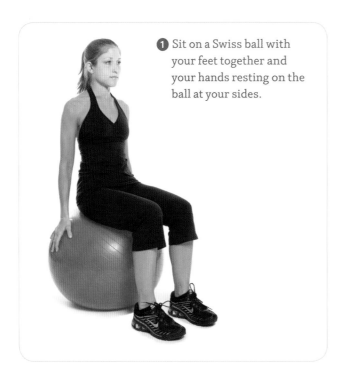

1 Sit on a Swiss ball with your feet together and your hands resting on the ball at your sides.

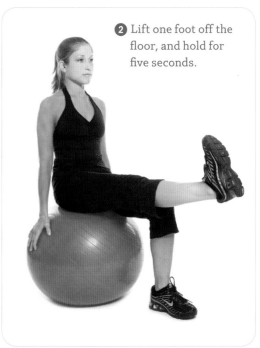

2 Lift one foot off the floor, and hold for five seconds.

QUICK GUIDE

TARGET
• Abdominals
• Quadriceps

TYPE
• Strengthening/stability

LEVEL
• Beginner

BENEFITS
• Stabilizes core
• Strengthens abdominals

NOT ADVISABLE IF YOU HAVE
• Neck issues
• Lower-back pain

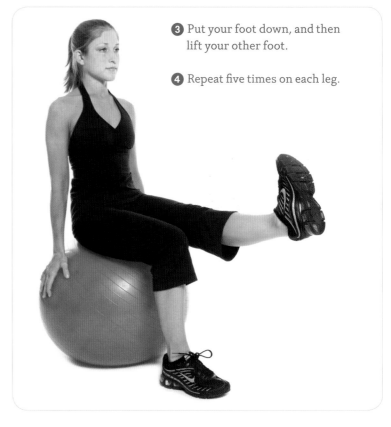

3 Put your foot down, and then lift your other foot.

4 Repeat five times on each leg.

BEST FOR

- rectus abdominis
- transversus abdominis
- rectus femoris
- vastus lateralis
- vastus intermedius
- vastus medialis

DO IT RIGHT

DO
- Sit up straight, and keep your abdominals activated.

AVOID
- Leaning forward as you lift your leg.

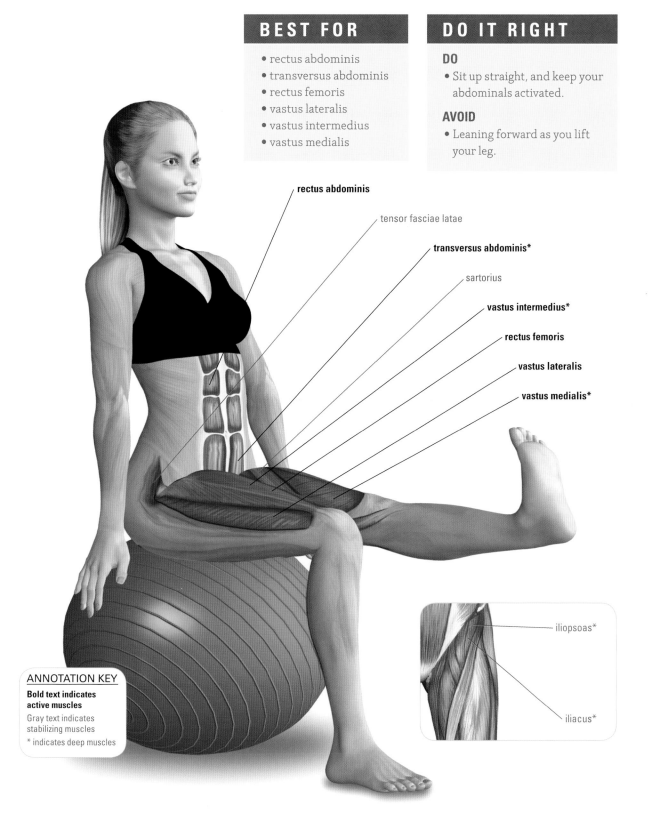

rectus abdominis

tensor fasciae latae

transversus abdominis*

sartorius

vastus intermedius*

rectus femoris

vastus lateralis

vastus medialis*

iliopsoas*

iliacus*

ANNOTATION KEY

Bold text indicates active muscles

Gray text indicates stabilizing muscles

* indicates deep muscles

STANDING STABILITY

CORE

1 Stand on a foam block, balancing on your left leg with your right knee bent. Extend both arms out to the side, parallel to the floor.

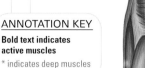

ANNOTATION KEY

Bold text indicates active muscles

* indicates deep muscles

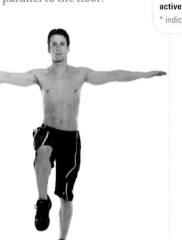

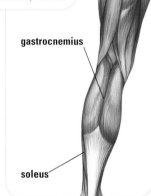

gluteus medius*

gastrocnemius

soleus

QUICK GUIDE

TARGET
• Abdominals
• Gluteal muscles
• Inner hip muscles

TYPE
• Stability/balance

LEVEL
• Beginner

BENEFITS
• Stabilizes core
• Improves balance

NOT ADVISABLE IF YOU HAVE
• Vestibular deficits

2 Close your eyes as you try to maintain your balance on the block.

3 Open your eyes, and then repeat, balancing on the right leg.

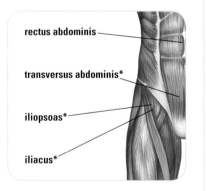

rectus abdominis

transversus abdominis*

iliopsoas*

iliacus*

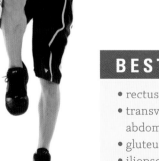

DO IT RIGHT

DO
• Open your eyes if you feel yourself tipping over.
• Keep your raised knee parallel to the floor.

AVOID
• Sloping your shoulders—your arms should form a straight line from shoulder to fingertips.

BEST FOR

• rectus abdominis
• transversus abdominis
• gluteus medius
• iliopsoas
• iliacus
• gastrocnemius
• soleus

STANDING EXTENSION

BEST FOR

- rectus abdominis
- transversus abdominis
- erector spinae
- multifidus spinae
- pectoralis major
- pectoralis minor

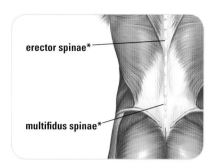

erector spinae*

multifidus spinae*

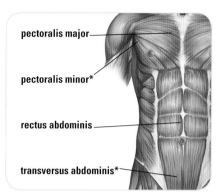

pectoralis major

pectoralis minor*

rectus abdominis

transversus abdominis*

1 Stand straight with your weight equally distributed between your feet. Place your hands on your hips.

ANNOTATION KEY
Bold text indicates active muscles
* indicates deep muscles

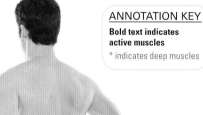

DO IT RIGHT

DO
- Keep your abdominals activated.

AVOID
- Hunching your shoulders.

2 Arch backward as far as you can comfortably go.

3 Return to the starting position, and repeat ten times.

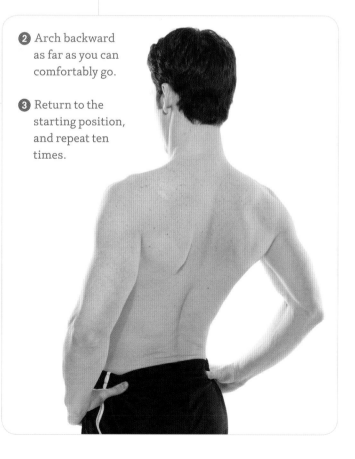

QUICK GUIDE

TARGET
- Abdominals
- Lower back

TYPE
- Stability

LEVEL
- Beginner

BENEFITS
- Stabilizes core
- Strengthens lower back

NOT ADVISABLE IF YOU HAVE
- Neck issues
- Lower-back pain

BASIC CRUNCH

CORE

1 Lie supine on the floor with your knees bent and your arms relaxed at your sides.

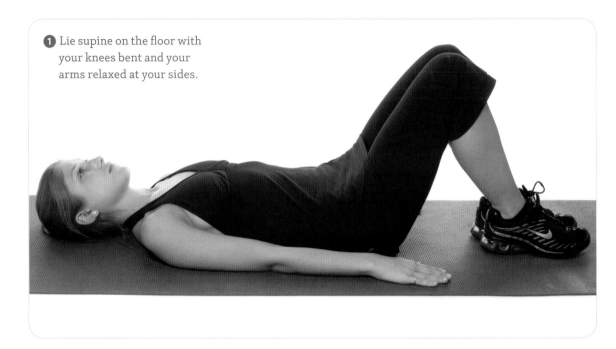

2 Clasp your hands behind your head. Keeping your elbows wide, engage the abdominals, and lift your upper torso to achieve a crunching movement.

3 Slowly return to the starting position. Repeat fifteen times for two sets.

BEST FOR

- rectus abdominis
- obliquus internus
- obliquus externus
- transversus abdominis

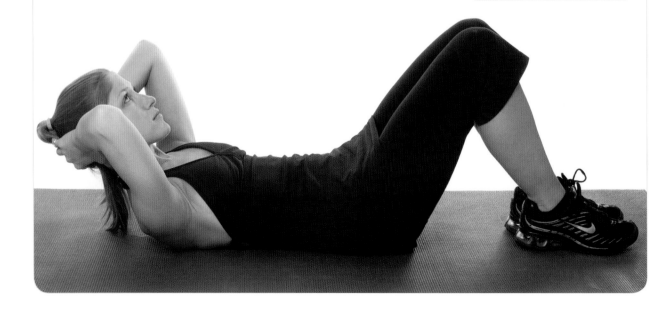

QUICK GUIDE

TARGET
• Abdominals

TYPE
• Strengthening

LEVEL
• Beginner

BENEFITS
• Strengthens the torso
• Improves pelvic and core
  stability

NOT ADVISABLE IF YOU HAVE
• Back pain
• Neck pain

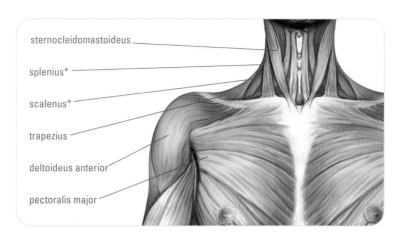

sternocleidomastoideus
splenius*
scalenus*
trapezius
deltoideus anterior
pectoralis major

ANNOTATION KEY
**Bold text indicates
active muscles**
Gray text indicates
stabilizing muscles
* indicates deep muscles

DO IT RIGHT

DO
• Initiate the movement with your
  abdominals.
• Keep your pelvis in the neutral position
  during the crunching motion.
• Tuck your chin slightly, directing your
  gaze toward the ceiling.

AVOID
• Pulling from the neck.
• Raising up more than 25 degrees.

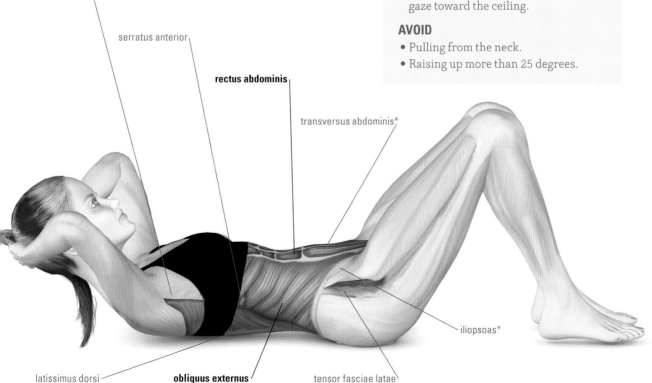

coracobrachialis

serratus anterior

rectus abdominis

transversus abdominis*

iliopsoas*

latissimus dorsi

obliquus externus

tensor fasciae latae

ABDOMINAL KICK

CORE

1 Lie supine on the floor with your knees bent. Pull your right knee toward your chest and straighten your left leg, raising it about 45 degrees from the floor.

2 Place your right hand on your right ankle, and your left hand on your right knee (this maintains proper alignment of leg).

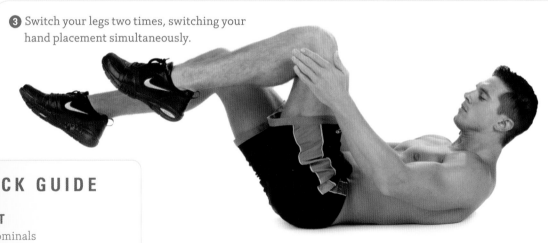

3 Switch your legs two times, switching your hand placement simultaneously.

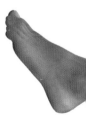

QUICK GUIDE

TARGET
• Abdominals

TYPE
• Strengthening

LEVEL
• Beginner

BENEFITS
• Strengthens abdominals
• Stabilizes core while extremities are in motion

NOT ADVISABLE IF YOU HAVE
• Neck issues
• Lower-back pain

DO IT RIGHT

DO
• Place your outside hand on the ankle of your bent leg, and your inside hand on your bent knee.
• Lift the top of your sternum forward.

AVOID
• Allowing your lower back to rise off the floor; use your abdominals to stabilize your core while switching legs.

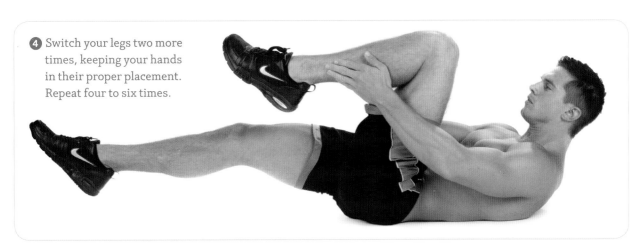

4 Switch your legs two more times, keeping your hands in their proper placement. Repeat four to six times.

BEST FOR

- rectus abdominis
- transversus abdominis
- obliquus internus
- biceps femoris
- triceps brachii
- biceps brachii
- tibialis anterior
- tensor fasciae latae

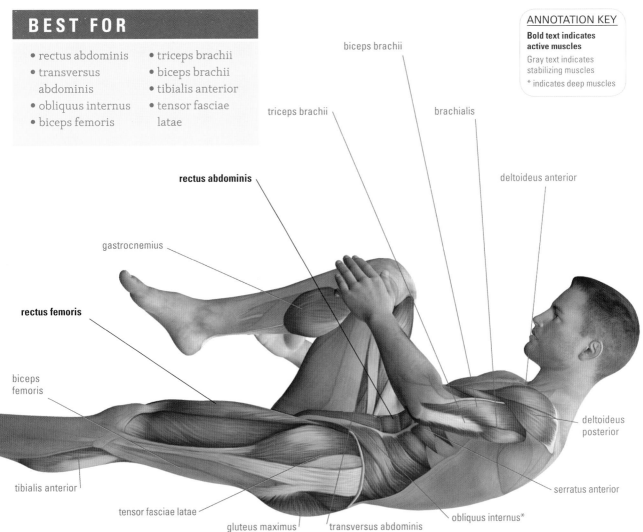

biceps brachii

triceps brachii

brachialis

deltoideus anterior

rectus abdominis

gastrocnemius

rectus femoris

biceps femoris

deltoideus posterior

tibialis anterior

serratus anterior

tensor fasciae latae

gluteus maximus

transversus abdominis

obliquus internus*

HALF CURL

CORE

1 Lie supine on the floor with your knees bent and arms straight by your sides.

Squeeze your legs together and keep your feet flat on the floor.

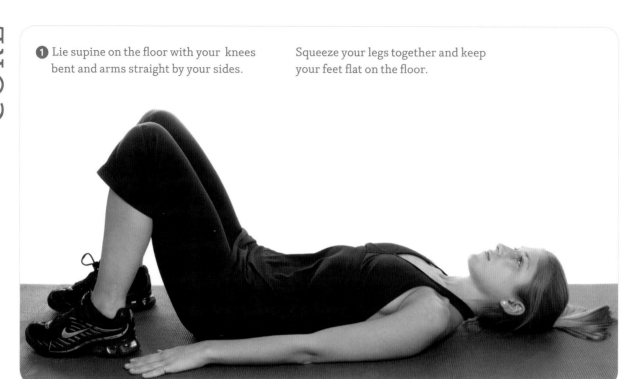

2 Using your upper abdominals, curl your upper back and shoulders off the mat. Keep your arms parallel to the floor and your lower back on the mat.

3 Hold for ten seconds. Return to the starting position, and repeat ten times.

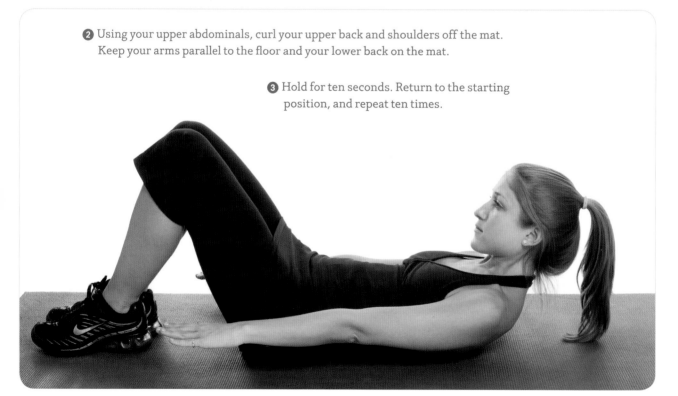

QUICK GUIDE

TARGET
- Upper abdominals

TYPE
- Strengthening

LEVEL
- Beginner

BENEFITS
- Strengthens core muscles
- Increases abdominal endurance

NOT ADVISABLE IF YOU HAVE
- Cervical spine issues

BEST FOR

- rectus abdominis
- latissimus dorsi
- pectoralis major
- sternohyoideus
- sternocleidomastoideus
- deltoideus medialis
- biceps brachii
- triceps brachii

DO IT RIGHT

DO
- Keep your arms parallel to the floor.

AVOID
- Curling your neck too far forward.
- Allowing your feet to raise off the floor.
- Raising up too far.

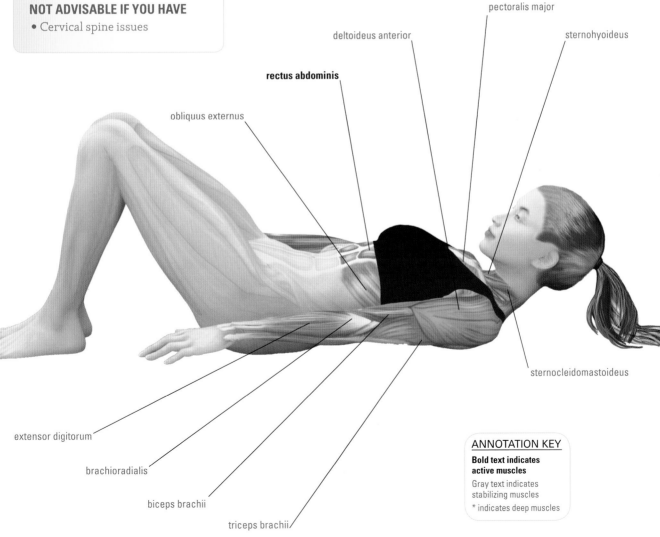

pectoralis major

deltoideus anterior

sternohyoideus

rectus abdominis

obliquus externus

sternocleidomastoideus

extensor digitorum

brachioradialis

biceps brachii

triceps brachii

ANNOTATION KEY

Bold text indicates active muscles

Gray text indicates stabilizing muscles

* indicates deep muscles

PRONE TRUNK RAISE

CORE

1. Lie prone on the floor. Bend your elbows, placing your hands flat on the floor on either side of your chest. Keep your elbows pulled in toward your body. Separate your legs hip-width apart, and extend through your toes. The tops of your feet should be touching the floor.

2. Inhale, and press against the floor with your hands and the tops of your feet, lifting your torso and hips off the floor. Contract your thighs, and tuck your tailbone toward your pubis.

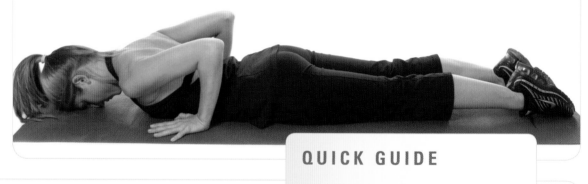

3. Lift through the top of your chest, fully extending your arms and creating an arch in your back from your upper torso. Push your shoulders down and back, and elongate your neck as you gaze slightly upward.

4. Hold for fifteen to thirty seconds, and exhale as you lower yourself to the floor.

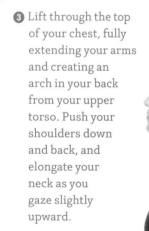

QUICK GUIDE

TARGET
- Abdominals
- Back

TYPE
- Strengthening/stability

LEVEL
- Beginner

BENEFITS
- Strengthens spine, arms, and wrists
- Stretches chest and abdominals
- Improves posture

NOT ADVISABLE IF YOU HAVE
- Back injury
- Wrist injury or carpal tunnel syndrome

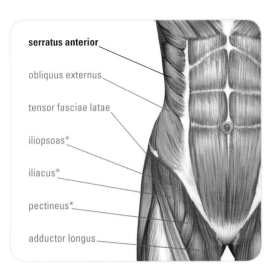

serratus anterior
obliquus externus
tensor fasciae latae
iliopsoas*
iliacus*
pectineus*
adductor longus

BEST FOR

- rhomboideus
- teres major
- teres minor
- trapezius
- latissimus dorsi
- erector spinae
- quadratus lumborum
- gluteus maximus
- pectoralis major
- serratus anterior
- rectus abdominis
- triceps brachii

DO IT RIGHT

DO
- Elongate your legs and arms to create full extension.
- Make sure that your wrists are positioned directly below your shoulders so that you do not exert too much pressure on your lower back.

AVOID
- Lifting your shoulders up toward your ears.
- Hyperextending your elbows.
- Jutting your rib cage out of your chest.
- Dropping your thighs.

ANNOTATION KEY
Bold text indicates active muscles
Gray text indicates stabilizing muscles
* indicates deep muscles

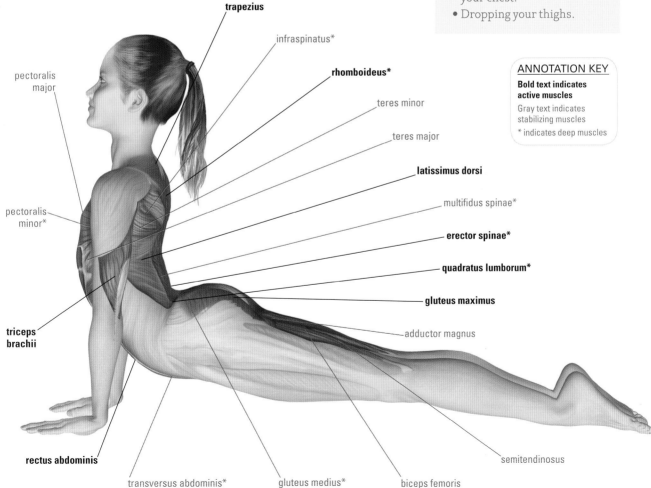

trapezius
infraspinatus*
rhomboideus*
teres minor
teres major
latissimus dorsi
multifidus spinae*
erector spinae*
quadratus lumborum*
gluteus maximus
adductor magnus
pectoralis major
pectoralis minor*
triceps brachii
rectus abdominis
transversus abdominis*
gluteus medius*
biceps femoris
semitendinosus

SEATED PIRIFORMIS STRETCH

CORE

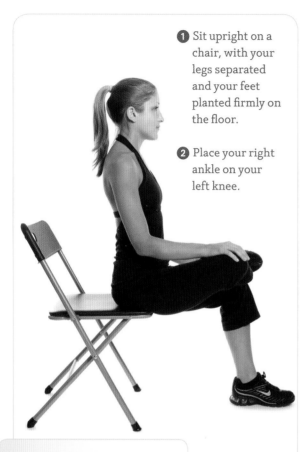

1 Sit upright on a chair, with your legs separated and your feet planted firmly on the floor.

2 Place your right ankle on your left knee.

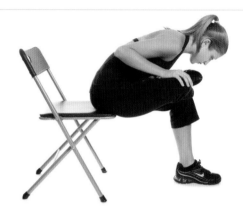

3 Lean forward from the hips until you feel a stretch in your buttocks and lower back. Push down on your right knee, and pull up on your right ankle, using the opposite knee as a fulcrum.

4 Return to the starting position, and repeat with your left leg crossed over the right.

MODIFICATION
More difficult:
Follow steps 1 though 3, and then bend forward more deeply.

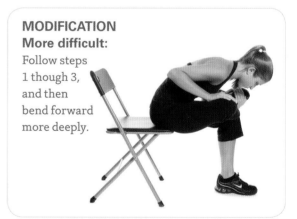

QUICK GUIDE

TARGET
• Piriformis
• Gluteal muscles

TYPE
• Flexibility

LEVEL
• Beginner

BENEFITS
• Stretches and strengthens the gluteal muscles
• Stretches the lower back

NOT ADVISABLE IF YOU HAVE
• Neck issues
• Lower-back pain

DO IT RIGHT

DO
• Bend only as far as is comfortable.

AVOID
• Allowing your buttocks to rise from the chair as you lean forward.

BEST FOR

• piriformis
• gluteus maximus
• gluteus medius
• gluteus minimus
• erector spinae
• quadratus femoris

PIRIFORMIS STRETCH

1 Lie supine on the floor with your knees bent.

2 Bring your left ankle over your right knee, resting it on your thigh. Place both hands around your right thigh.

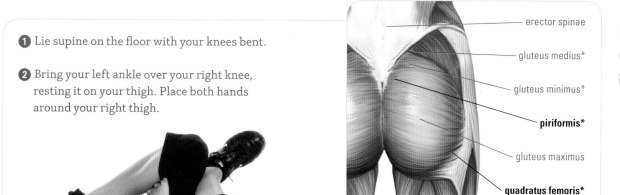

- erector spinae
- gluteus medius*
- gluteus minimus*
- **piriformis***
- gluteus maximus
- **quadratus femoris***

ANNOTATION KEY
Bold text indicates active muscles
Gray text indicates stabilizing muscles
* indicates deep muscles

3 Gently pull your right thigh toward your chest until you feel the stretch in your buttocks. Hold for fifteen seconds and then switch sides. Repeat sequence with your left leg crossed over your right.

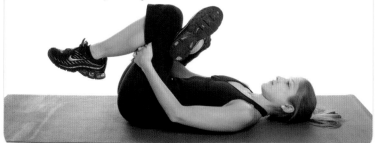

QUICK GUIDE

TARGET
- Piriformis
- Gluteal muscles

TYPE
- Flexibility

LEVEL
- Intermediate

BENEFITS
- Stretches and strengthens the piriformis and gluteal muscles

NOT ADVISABLE IF YOU HAVE
- Hip dysfunction

DO IT RIGHT

DO
- Relax your hips so that you can go deeper into the stretch.

AVOID
- Rushing the stretch.

BEST FOR

- piriformis
- gluteus maximus
- gluteus medius
- gluteus minimus
- erector spinae
- quadratus femoris

RUSSIAN TWIST

CORE

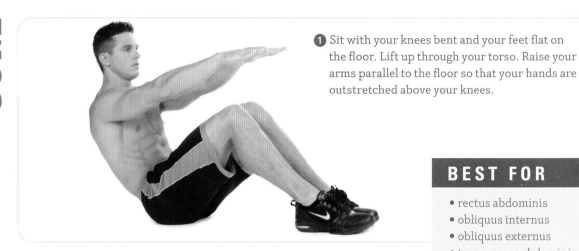

1 Sit with your knees bent and your feet flat on the floor. Lift up through your torso. Raise your arms parallel to the floor so that your hands are outstretched above your knees.

BEST FOR

- rectus abdominis
- obliquus internus
- obliquus externus
- transversus abdominis
- vastus intermedius
- rectus femoris
- iliacus
- iliopsoas

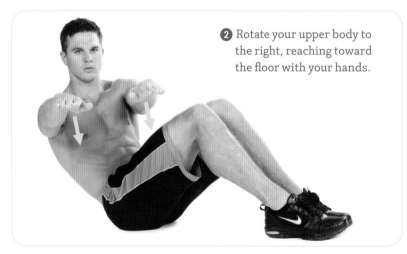

2 Rotate your upper body to the right, reaching toward the floor with your hands.

QUICK GUIDE

TARGET
- Abdominals
- Hip flexors
- Quadriceps

TYPE
- Strengthening

LEVEL
- Intermediate

BENEFITS
- Increases abdominal endurance
- Strengthens hip flexors

NOT ADVISABLE IF YOU HAVE
- Neck issues
- Lower-back pain

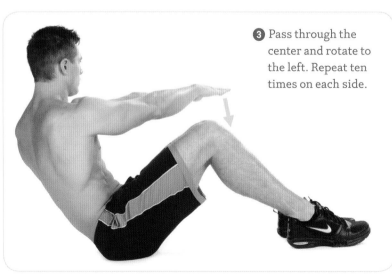

3 Pass through the center and rotate to the left. Repeat ten times on each side.

MODIFICATION

More difficult: Lift your feet off the floor, and rotate your torso from side to side, pulling your knees in and out as you twist.

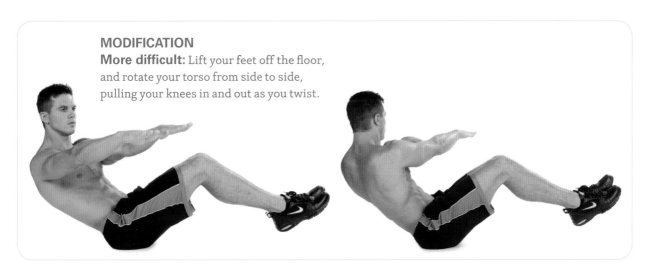

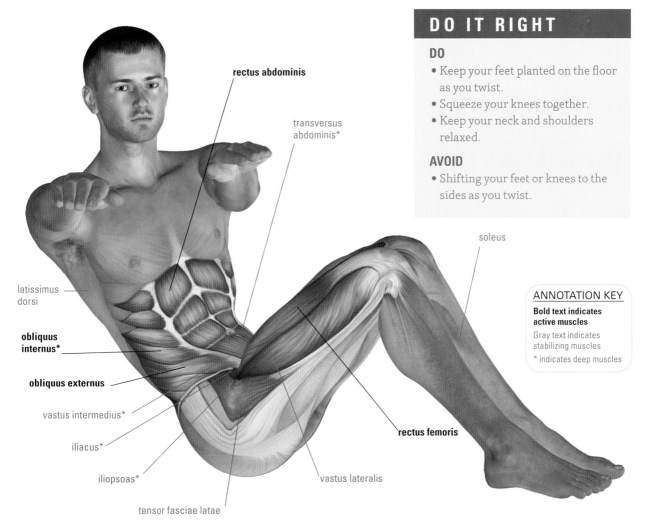

rectus abdominis

transversus abdominis*

latissimus dorsi

obliquus internus*

obliquus externus

vastus intermedius*

iliacus*

iliopsoas*

tensor fasciae latae

vastus lateralis

rectus femoris

soleus

DO IT RIGHT

DO
- Keep your feet planted on the floor as you twist.
- Squeeze your knees together.
- Keep your neck and shoulders relaxed.

AVOID
- Shifting your feet or knees to the sides as you twist.

ANNOTATION KEY
Bold text indicates active muscles

Gray text indicates stabilizing muscles

* indicates deep muscles

LOW CURL-UP

CORE

1 Lie supine on the floor with your legs straight and your arms outstretched to the sides. Your spine should be in a neutral position.

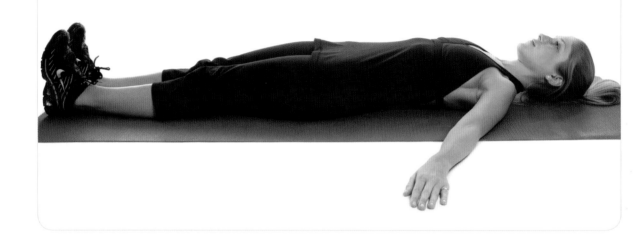

2 Tighten your abdominals, and without flattening or bending your lower back, curl up your upper body by raising your head and shoulders off the floor.

3 Hold for two seconds. Return to the starting position, and repeat ten times.

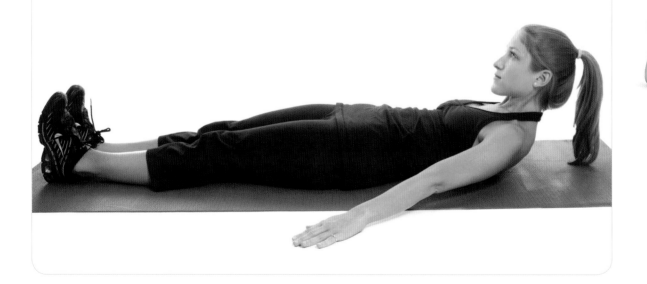

QUICK GUIDE

TARGET
- Lower abdominals
- Neck muscles

TYPE
- Strengthening

LEVEL
- Intermediate

BENEFITS
- Stabilizes core
- Strengthens abdominals

NOT ADVISABLE IF YOU HAVE
- Neck issues
- Lower-back pain

BEST FOR

- rectus abdominis
- transversus abdominis
- pectoralis major
- sternohyoideus
- sternocleidomastoideus
- deltoideus medialis
- trapezius

DO IT RIGHT

DO
- Curl up without bending your neck if you feel any pain.

AVOID
- Bending your knees as you lift your shoulders.

ANNOTATION KEY
Bold text indicates active muscles
Gray text indicates stabilizing muscles
* indicates deep muscles

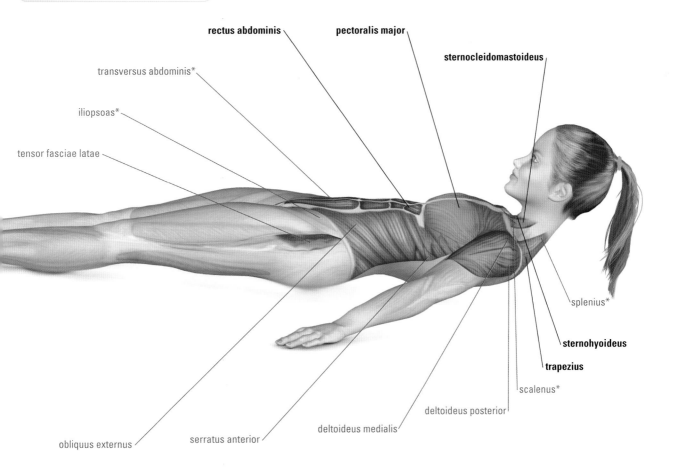

rectus abdominis · pectoralis major · sternocleidomastoideus · transversus abdominis* · iliopsoas* · tensor fasciae latae · splenius* · sternohyoideus · trapezius · scalenus* · deltoideus posterior · deltoideus medialis · serratus anterior · obliquus externus

REVERSE BRIDGE ROTATION

CORE

❶ Lie supine with your shoulders and lower back on a Swiss ball and your feet hip-width apart. Your knees should be bent at 90 degrees.

❷ Pick up a medicine ball with both hands, and position your arms straight up.

❸ Rotate your upper body to the left, rolling onto your left shoulder on top of the Swiss ball.

❹ Hold for five seconds, and then slowly roll back to the starting position with the Swiss ball in the center of your shoulders.

BEST FOR

- obliquus externus
- obliquus internus

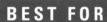

QUICK GUIDE

TARGET
- Obliques
- Abdominals

TYPE
- Strengthening/stability

LEVEL
- Intermediate

BENEFITS
- Stabilizes core
- Strengthens obliques and abdominals

NOT ADVISABLE IF YOU HAVE
- Neck issues
- Lower-back pain

❺ Repeat the exercise, rotating your torso and rolling your shoulders to the right.

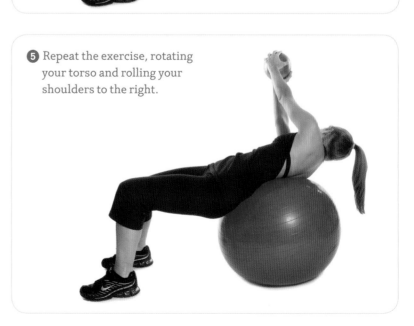

DO IT RIGHT

DO

- Position the Swiss ball directly between your shoulder blades to start the exercise.
- Activate your abdominals so that you maintain neutral alignment.
- Keep your hips in line with your knees as you rotate your upper body, to work your spinal rotators.

AVOID

- Bending your arms.
- Continuing to rotate the Swiss ball when it is lying directly under one shoulder and both shoulders are vertical.

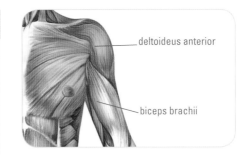

deltoideus anterior

biceps brachii

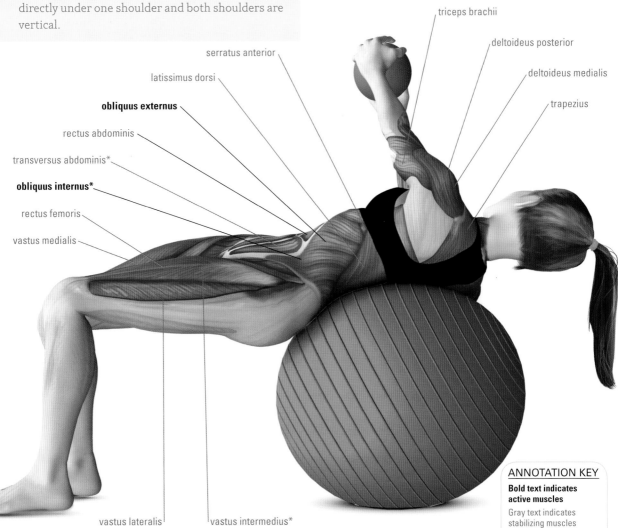

serratus anterior

latissimus dorsi

obliquus externus

rectus abdominis

transversus abdominis*

obliquus internus*

rectus femoris

vastus medialis

triceps brachii

deltoideus posterior

deltoideus medialis

trapezius

vastus lateralis

vastus intermedius*

ANNOTATION KEY

Bold text indicates active muscles

Gray text indicates stabilizing muscles

* indicates deep muscles

REVERSE BRIDGE BALL ROLL

CORE

1 Lie supine with your lower back on a Swiss ball and your feet together. Your knees should be bent at 90 degrees. Position your arms out to the sides.

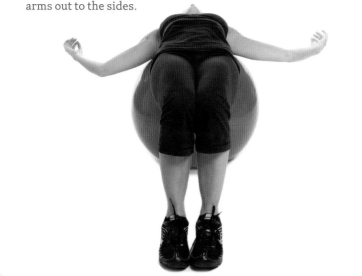

DO IT RIGHT

DO
• Exhale as you roll on the ball, and inhale as you return to the starting position.
• Hold your body stable as you roll across the ball, working against the ball's natural rotation.
• Increase the space between your feet if necessary to maintain your balance.

AVOID
• Allowing your pelvis to drop out of alignment— your body should form a straight line from your shoulders to your knees.
• Continuing to rotate the ball when it is lying directly under one shoulder and both shoulders are vertical.

2 Move your upper body across the ball to the left, rolling the ball under your shoulders and toward your left shoulder.

3 Hold for five seconds, and then slowly roll the ball back to the center of your shoulders.

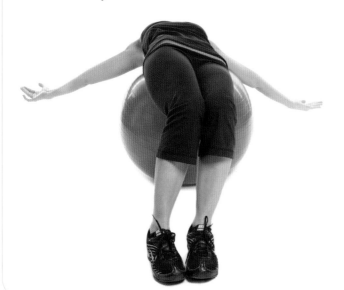

4 Return to the starting position, and then roll to the right. Repeat five times on each side.

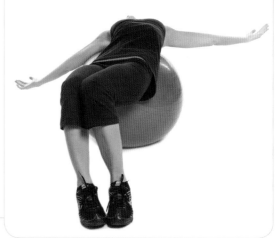

QUICK GUIDE

TARGET
- Obliques
- Abdominals

TYPE
- Strengthening/stability

LEVEL
- Intermediate

BENEFITS
- Stabilizes core
- Strengthens obliques and abdominals

NOT ADVISABLE IF YOU HAVE
- Severe neck pain
- Severe lower-back pain

MODIFICATION
Easier: Rather than keeping your feet together, position them about shoulder-width apart. Then follow steps 2 through 4.

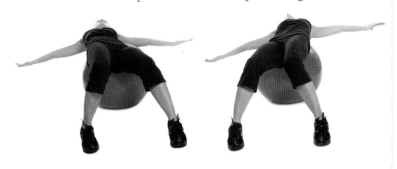

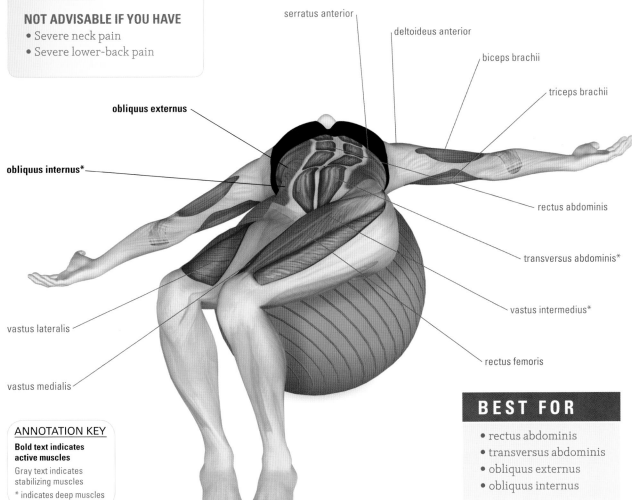

serratus anterior

deltoideus anterior

biceps brachii

triceps brachii

obliquus externus

obliquus internus*

rectus abdominis

transversus abdominis*

vastus intermedius*

vastus lateralis

rectus femoris

vastus medialis

ANNOTATION KEY
Bold text indicates active muscles
Gray text indicates stabilizing muscles
* indicates deep muscles

BEST FOR
- rectus abdominis
- transversus abdominis
- obliquus externus
- obliquus internus

MEDICINE BALL AB CURLS

CORE

QUICK GUIDE

TARGET
• Abdominals

TYPE
• Strengthening/stability

LEVEL
• Intermediate

BENEFITS
• Strengthens abdominals

NOT ADVISABLE IF YOU HAVE
• Severe neck pain
• Severe lower-back pain

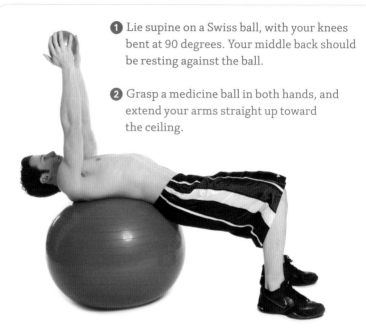

❶ Lie supine on a Swiss ball, with your knees bent at 90 degrees. Your middle back should be resting against the ball.

❷ Grasp a medicine ball in both hands, and extend your arms straight up toward the ceiling.

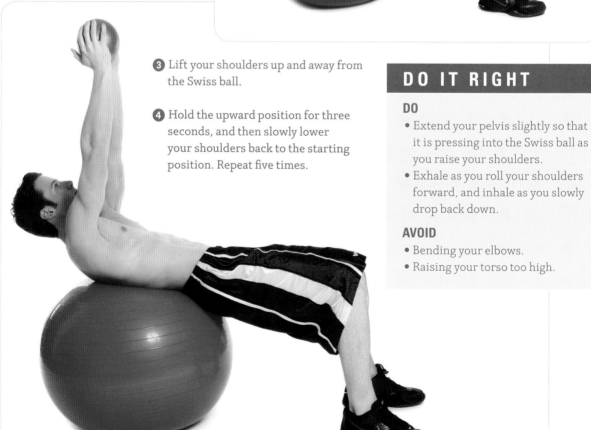

❸ Lift your shoulders up and away from the Swiss ball.

❹ Hold the upward position for three seconds, and then slowly lower your shoulders back to the starting position. Repeat five times.

DO IT RIGHT

DO
• Extend your pelvis slightly so that it is pressing into the Swiss ball as you raise your shoulders.
• Exhale as you roll your shoulders forward, and inhale as you slowly drop back down.

AVOID
• Bending your elbows.
• Raising your torso too high.

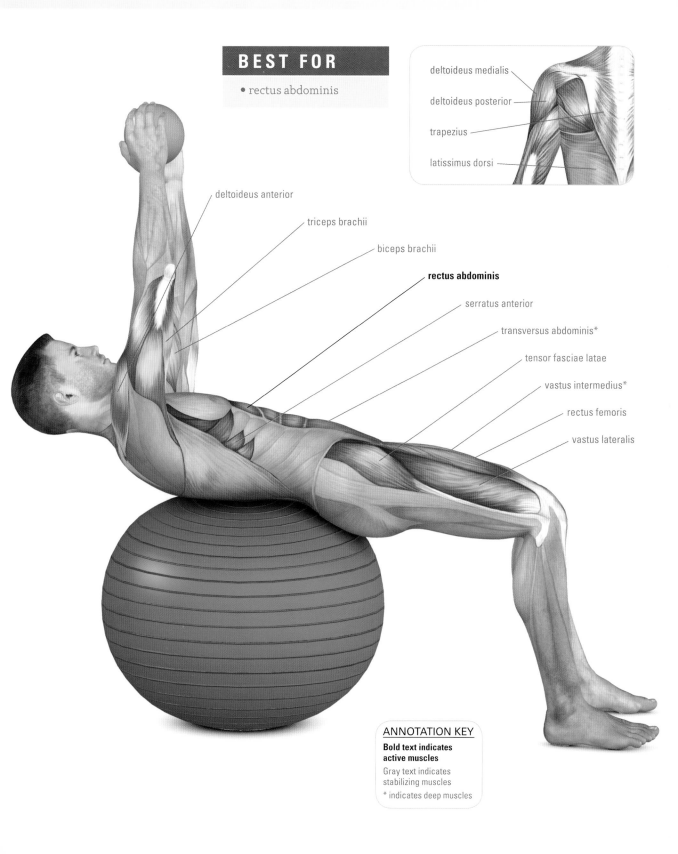

BEST FOR

• rectus abdominis

deltoideus medialis

deltoideus posterior

trapezius

latissimus dorsi

deltoideus anterior

triceps brachii

biceps brachii

rectus abdominis

serratus anterior

transversus abdominis*

tensor fasciae latae

vastus intermedius*

rectus femoris

vastus lateralis

ANNOTATION KEY

Bold text indicates active muscles

Gray text indicates stabilizing muscles

* indicates deep muscles

PLANK ROLL-DOWN

CORE

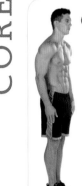

1 Stand straight with your weight equally distributed between your feet.

2 Relaxing your neck, bend from your waist and bring your hands down toward the floor. Place them in front of your feet so that they are flat on the floor.

DO IT RIGHT

DO
- Keep your spine and legs straight.
- Move slowly and steadily.
- Make sure that your abdominals remain up and in.

AVOID
- Bending your knees or spine.
- Allowing your elbows to bend.

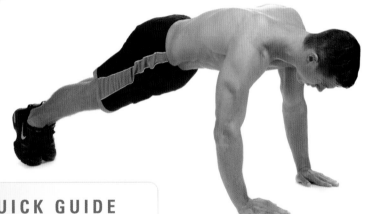

3 Walk your hands away from your feet until your body reaches a plank position, forming a straight line from your shoulders to your heels.

QUICK GUIDE

TARGET
- Abdominals
- Pectoral muscles
- Upper-arm muscles

TYPE
- Strengthening/stability

LEVEL
- Intermediate

BENEFITS
- Stabilizes core
- Strengthens abdominals

NOT ADVISABLE IF YOU HAVE
- Wrist pain
- Shoulder issues
- Lower-back pain

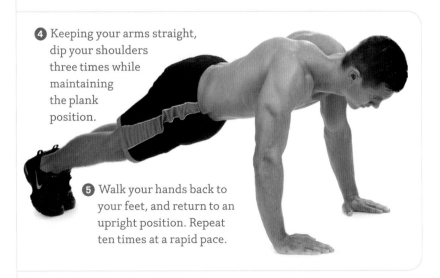

4 Keeping your arms straight, dip your shoulders three times while maintaining the plank position.

5 Walk your hands back to your feet, and return to an upright position. Repeat ten times at a rapid pace.

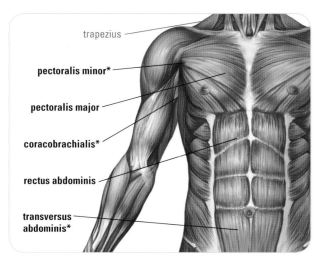

- trapezius
- **pectoralis minor***
- **pectoralis major**
- **coracobrachialis***
- **rectus abdominis**
- **transversus abdominis***

MODIFICATION

Easier: Roll down to a plank position on your elbows, rather than on your hands. Supporting your torso with your forearms and maintaining the plank position, dip up and down three times.

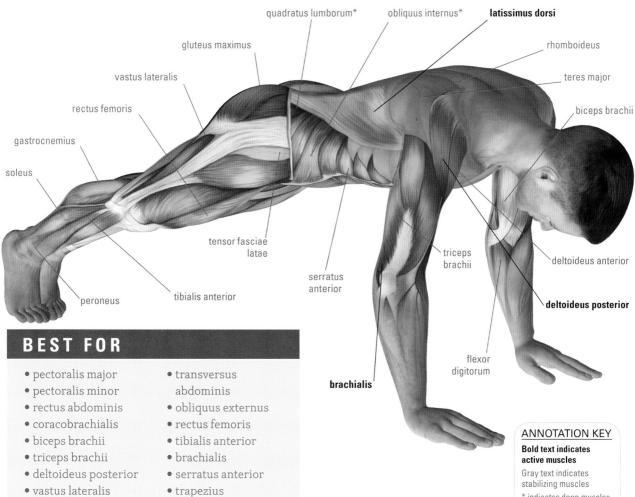

- quadratus lumborum*
- obliquus internus*
- **latissimus dorsi**
- gluteus maximus
- rhomboideus
- vastus lateralis
- teres major
- rectus femoris
- biceps brachii
- gastrocnemius
- soleus
- tensor fasciae latae
- triceps brachii
- deltoideus anterior
- serratus anterior
- **deltoideus posterior**
- peroneus
- tibialis anterior
- flexor digitorum
- **brachialis**

BEST FOR

- pectoralis major
- pectoralis minor
- rectus abdominis
- coracobrachialis
- biceps brachii
- triceps brachii
- deltoideus posterior
- vastus lateralis
- transversus abdominis
- obliquus externus
- rectus femoris
- tibialis anterior
- brachialis
- serratus anterior
- trapezius

ANNOTATION KEY

Bold text indicates active muscles

Gray text indicates stabilizing muscles

* indicates deep muscles

THE POINTER

CORE

① Begin on your hands and knees, with your wrists directly below your shoulders and your knees directly below your hips. Your fingertips should be facing forward with your hands shoulder-width apart. Gaze at the floor, keeping your head in a neutral position.

BEST FOR

- gluteus maximus
- biceps femoris
- gluteus medius
- deltoideus medialis
- adductor magnus
- rectus abdominis
- transversus abdominis
- obliquus internus
- tensor fasciae latae
- adductor longus
- rectus femoris

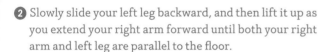

② Slowly slide your left leg backward, and then lift it up as you extend your right arm forward until both your right arm and left leg are parallel to the floor.

③ Hold for ten seconds, and return to the starting position.

④ Repeat with the opposite arm and leg.

⑤ Repeat the entire sequence on each side.

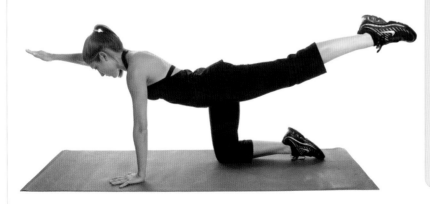

QUICK GUIDE

TARGET
- Core stability
- Pelvic stabilizers
- Hip extensor muscles
- Oblique muscles

TYPE
- Strengthening/stability

LEVEL
- Intermediate

BENEFITS
- Tones arms, legs, and abdominals

NOT ADVISABLE IF YOU HAVE
- Wrist pain
- Lower-back pain
- Knee pain while kneeling
- Inability to stabilize the spine while moving limbs

DO IT RIGHT

DO

- Keep your back flat throughout the exercise.

AVOID

- Tilting your pelvis during the movement—slide your leg along the surface of the floor before lifting.
- Allowing your back to sink into an arched position.

MODIFICATION

More difficult: Instead of kneeling, press into a plank position to begin, and then raise the opposite arm and leg.

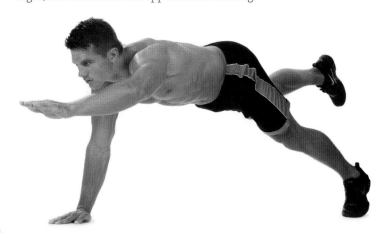

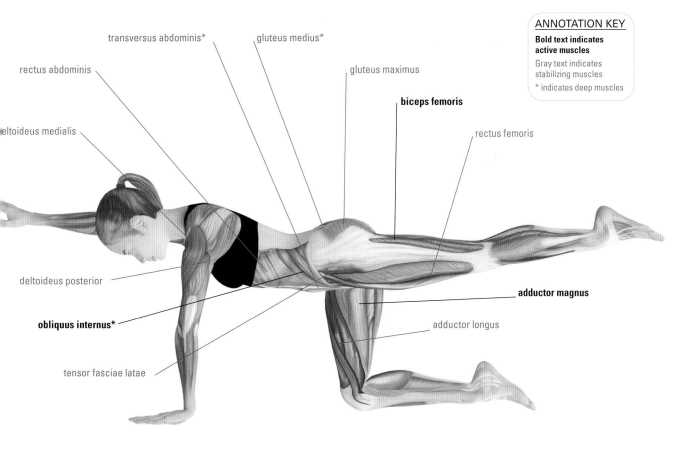

transversus abdominis*

gluteus medius*

rectus abdominis

gluteus maximus

biceps femoris

eltoideus medialis

rectus femoris

deltoideus posterior

adductor magnus

obliquus internus*

adductor longus

tensor fasciae latae

PLANK

CORE

❶ Lie supine on the mat, supporting your upper body on your forearms. Bend your legs, and rest your weight on your knees.

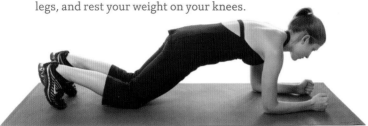

DO IT RIGHT

DO
• Lengthen through your neck.

AVOID
• Allowing your back to sag.
• Allowing your shoulders to collapse into your shoulder joints.

❷ Push through your forearms to bring your shoulders up toward the ceiling as you straighten your legs.

❸ With control, lower your shoulders until you feel them coming together in your back.

❹ Return to the starting position, and repeat five times.

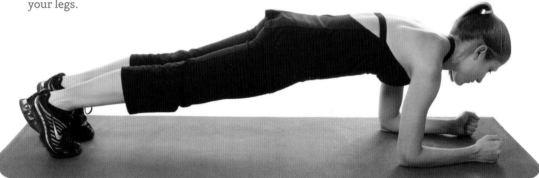

QUICK GUIDE

TARGET
• Scapular stabilizers
• Core muscles

TYPE
• Strengthening/stability

LEVEL
• Intermediate

BENEFITS
• Stabilizes core
• Strengthens abdominals

NOT ADVISABLE IF YOU HAVE
• Shoulder injury
• Intense back pain

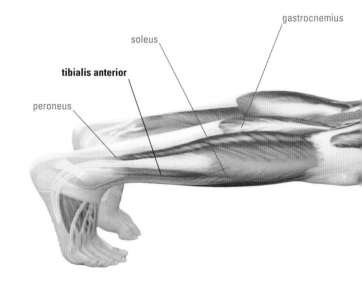

gastrocnemius

soleus

tibialis anterior

peroneus

MODIFICATION

Easier: Rather than using your forearms to support your upper body, straighten your arms, holding yourself up on your hands.

Then, push through your arms into a plank position.

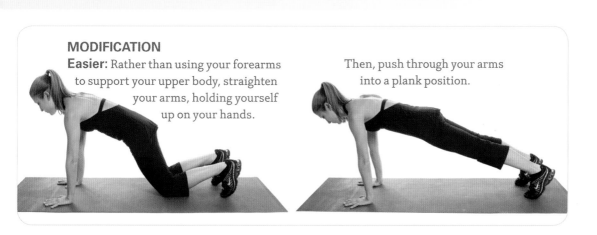

BEST FOR

- deltoideus
- rhomboideus
- rectus abdominis
- biceps brachii
- triceps brachii
- tensor fasciae latae
- rectus femoris
- transversus abdominis
- obliquus internus
- serratus anterior
- tibialis anterior

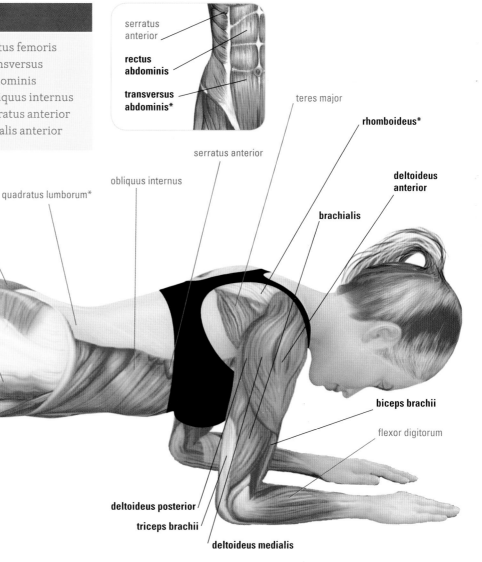

serratus anterior

rectus abdominis

transversus abdominis*

teres major

rhomboideus*

deltoideus anterior

serratus anterior

brachialis

gluteus maximus

quadratus lumborum*

obliquus internus

tensor fasciae latae

vastus lateralis

rectus femoris

biceps brachii

flexor digitorum

deltoideus posterior

triceps brachii

deltoideus medialis

ANNOTATION KEY

Bold text indicates active muscles

Gray text indicates stabilizing muscles

* indicates deep muscles

FRONT PLANK

CORE

1 Sit with your legs parallel and stretched out in front of you. Place your hands behind you with your fingers pointed toward your hips.

DO IT RIGHT

DO
- Keep your pelvis elevated throughout the exercise.

AVOID
- Allowing your shoulders to sink into their sockets. If your legs do not feel strong enough to support your body, slightly bend your knees.

2 Press up through your arms and lift your chest up, squeezing your buttocks and lifting your hips while pressing your heels into the floor. Continue lifting your pelvis until your body forms a long line from your shoulders to your feet.

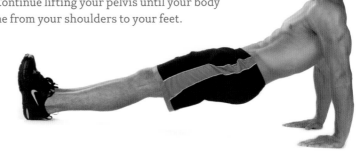

QUICK GUIDE

TARGET
- Hip extensor muscles
- Core stabilizers
- Arm muscles
- Leg muscles

TYPE
- Strengthening/stability

LEVEL
- Intermediate

BENEFITS
- Stabilizes core
- Strengthens abdominals

NOT ADVISABLE IF YOU HAVE
- Wrist pain
- Knee pain
- Shoulder injury
- Shooting pains down leg

3 Without allowing your pelvis to drop, raise your straightened right leg.

4 Slowly lower your leg to the floor, and switch to the left leg. Repeat four to six times on each side.

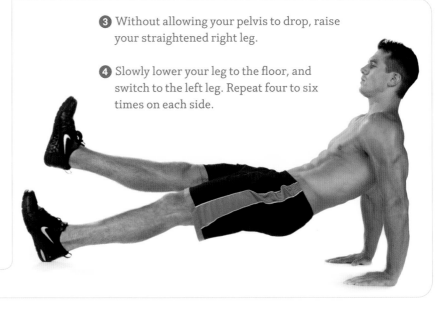

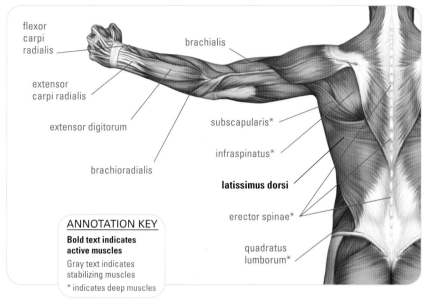

flexor
carpi
radialis

brachialis

extensor
carpi radialis

extensor digitorum

subscapularis*

infraspinatus*

brachioradialis

latissimus dorsi

erector spinae*

quadratus
lumborum*

ANNOTATION KEY

**Bold text indicates
active muscles**

Gray text indicates
stabilizing muscles

* indicates deep muscles

BEST FOR

- gluteus maximus
- biceps femoris
- deltoideus
- rectus femoris
- adductor magnus
- tensor fasciae latae
- rectus abdominis
- transversus abdominis
- adductor longus
- obliquus externus
- latissimus dorsi
- triceps brachii

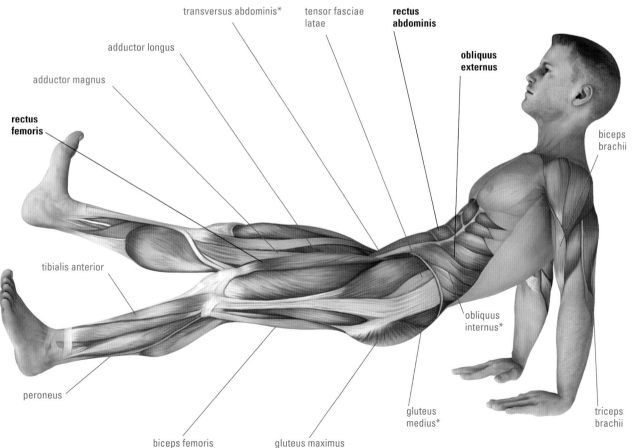

transversus abdominis*

tensor fasciae
latae

**rectus
abdominis**

adductor longus

**obliquus
externus**

adductor magnus

**rectus
femoris**

biceps
brachii

tibialis anterior

obliquus
internus*

peroneus

gluteus
medius*

triceps
brachii

biceps femoris

gluteus maximus

SIDE WALKING

CORE

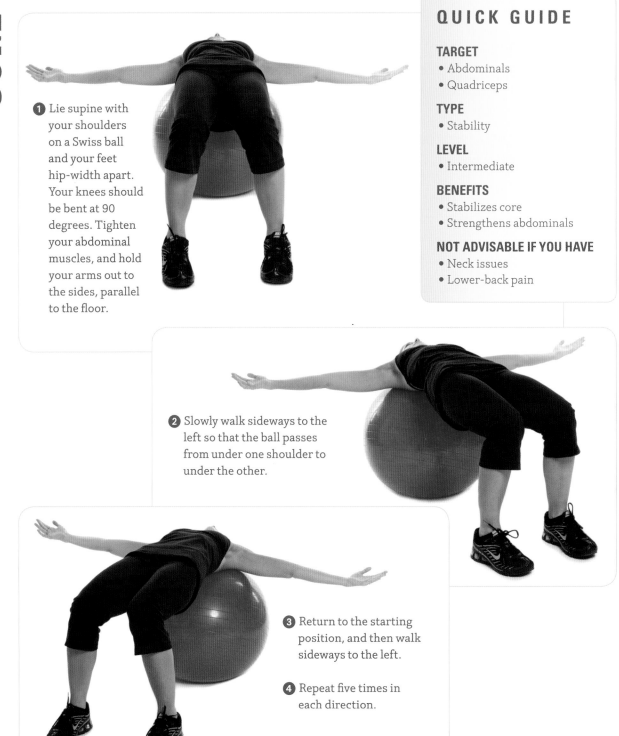

① Lie supine with your shoulders on a Swiss ball and your feet hip-width apart. Your knees should be bent at 90 degrees. Tighten your abdominal muscles, and hold your arms out to the sides, parallel to the floor.

② Slowly walk sideways to the left so that the ball passes from under one shoulder to under the other.

③ Return to the starting position, and then walk sideways to the left.

④ Repeat five times in each direction.

QUICK GUIDE

TARGET
• Abdominals
• Quadriceps

TYPE
• Stability

LEVEL
• Intermediate

BENEFITS
• Stabilizes core
• Strengthens abdominals

NOT ADVISABLE IF YOU HAVE
• Neck issues
• Lower-back pain

DO IT RIGHT

DO
- Activate your abdominals so that you maintain neutral alignment, with your body forming a straight line from shoulders to knees.

AVOID
- Allowing your pelvis to drop out of alignment.
- Lateral ball movement.

BEST FOR

- rectus abdominis
- transversus abdominis
- rectus femoris
- vastus lateralis
- vastus intermedius
- vastus medialis
- adductor brevis
- adductor longus
- adductor magnus
- tensor fasciae latae

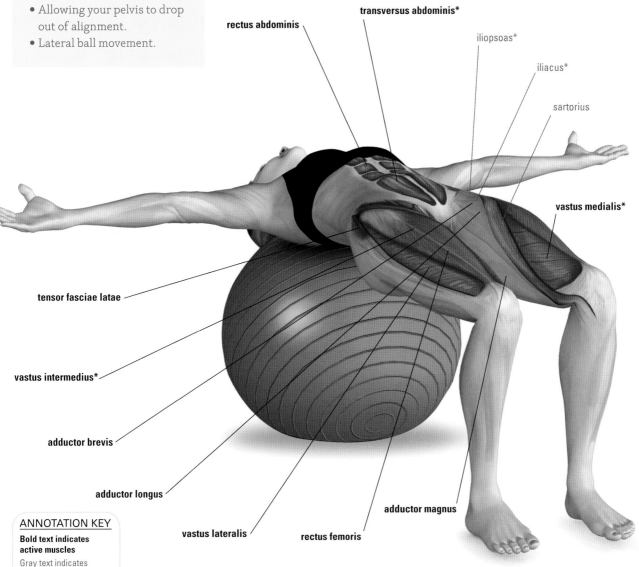

rectus abdominis

transversus abdominis*

iliopsoas*

iliacus*

sartorius

vastus medialis*

tensor fasciae latae

vastus intermedius*

adductor brevis

adductor longus

vastus lateralis

rectus femoris

adductor magnus

ANNOTATION KEY
Bold text indicates active muscles
Gray text indicates stabilizing muscles
* indicates deep muscles

JACKKNIFE

CORE

1 Place your hands on the floor, with your legs extended so that the tops of your feet rest on top of a Swiss ball. Keep your spine in a neutral position.

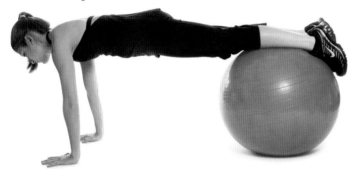

2 Flex your hips, and pull your knees up toward your chest, driving your hips toward the ceiling and retracting your abdomen.

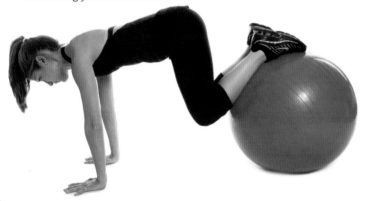

QUICK GUIDE

TARGET
• Abdominals
• Hip flexors

TYPE
• Strengthening/stability

LEVEL
• Advanced

BENEFITS
• Stabilizes core
• Strengthens abdominals
• Hip flexors

NOT ADVISABLE IF YOU HAVE
• Neck issues
• Lower-back pain

3 Continue to pull in until your buttocks are resting on top of your heels.

4 Hold for five seconds, and then extend your hips to straighten your legs and return to the starting position.

5 Repeat entire sequence three times.

BEST FOR

• iliacus
• iliopsoas
• obliquus externus
• obliquus internus
• rectus abdominis
• sartorius
• tibialis anterior
• transversus abdominis

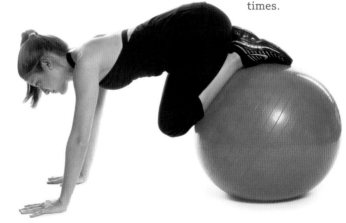

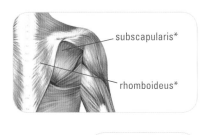

subscapularis*

rhomboideus*

ANNOTATION KEY

**Bold text indicates
active muscles**

Gray text indicates
stabilizing muscles

* indicates deep muscles

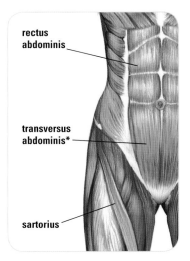

**rectus
abdominis**

**transversus
abdominis***

sartorius

DO IT RIGHT

DO

- Keep your chest high and retracted.
- Elongate your neck and extend your elbows throughout the movement.
- Position your hands on the floor so that they are directly below your shoulders.

AVOID

- Bending your elbows.
- Allowing your shoulders to elevate toward your ears.

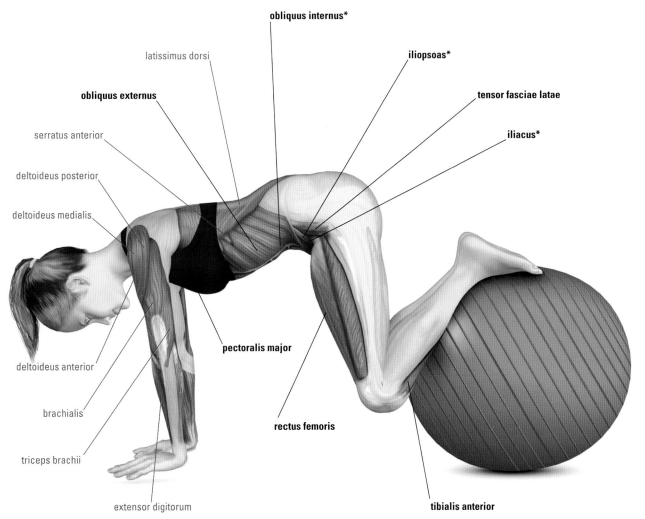

obliquus internus*

latissimus dorsi

obliquus externus

serratus anterior

deltoideus posterior

deltoideus medialis

deltoideus anterior

brachialis

triceps brachii

extensor digitorum

pectoralis major

rectus femoris

iliopsoas*

tensor fasciae latae

iliacus*

tibialis anterior

ROTATED BACK EXTENSION

CORE

① Lie prone on a Swiss ball, so that your navel is on the center of the ball. Extend your legs behind you, resting on your toes.

② Place your hands behind your head, with your elbows out.

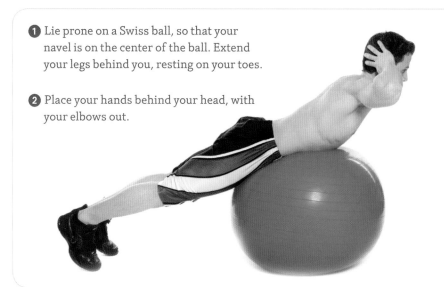

DO IT RIGHT

DO
- Keep your toes firmly planted on the floor.
- Keep your arms out at a 90-degree angle to your body with your elbows bent.
- Widen your feet for increased stability.

AVOID
- Shifting your hips as you rotate—hold them square to the ball throughout the movement.

QUICK GUIDE

TARGET
- Obliques
- Back

TYPE
- Strengthening/stability

LEVEL
- Advanced

BENEFITS
- Strengthens back muscles
- Strengthens obliques

NOT ADVISABLE IF YOU HAVE
- Neck issues
- Lower-back pain

③ Extend your back, lifting your chest away from the ball, and rotate your torso to the right.

④ Hold for five seconds, and then lower your chest and shoulders back to the starting position.

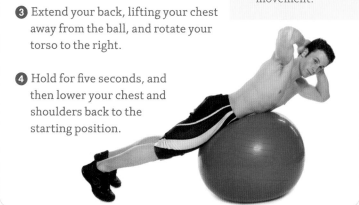

⑤ Repeat, extending your back and rotating your torso to the left. Repeat entire sequence three times in both directions.

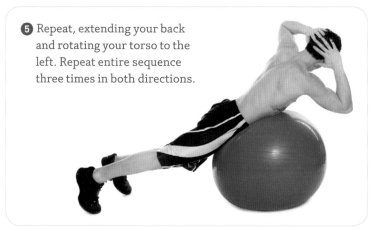

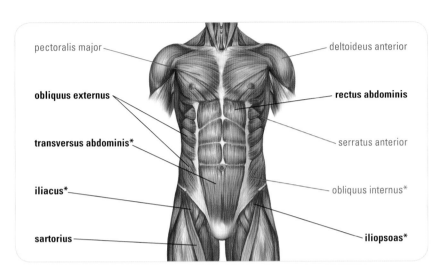

pectoralis major
deltoideus anterior
obliquus externus
rectus abdominis
transversus abdominis*
serratus anterior
iliacus*
obliquus internus*
sartorius
iliopsoas*

BEST FOR

- erector spinae
- obliquus externus

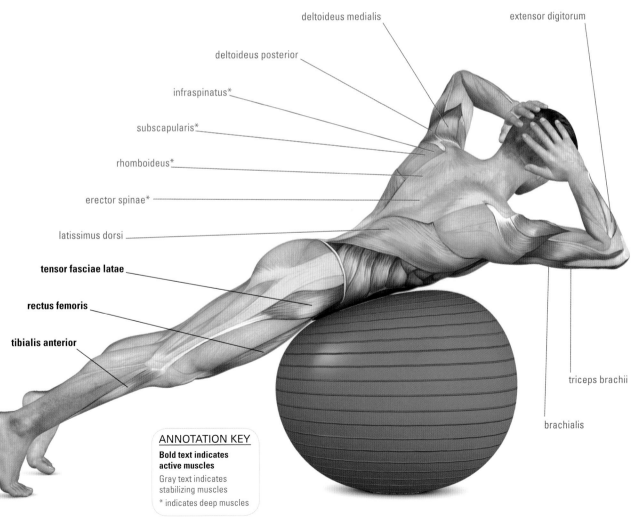

deltoideus medialis
extensor digitorum
deltoideus posterior
infraspinatus*
subscapularis*
rhomboideus*
erector spinae*
latissimus dorsi
tensor fasciae latae
rectus femoris
tibialis anterior
triceps brachii
brachialis

ANNOTATION KEY
Bold text indicates active muscles
Gray text indicates stabilizing muscles
* indicates deep muscles

TRANSVERSE ABS

CORE

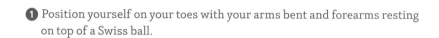

1 Position yourself on your toes with your arms bent and forearms resting on top of a Swiss ball.

2 Form a long, straight line from your ankles to your shoulders.

3 Hold this position for as long as you can.

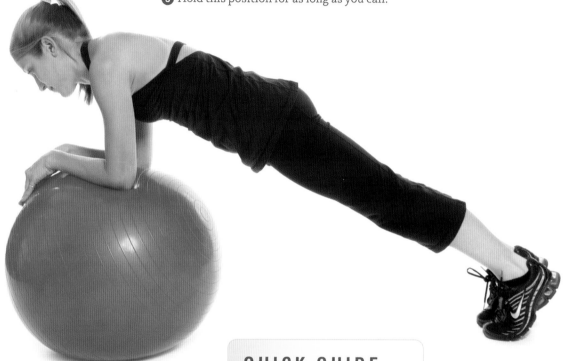

QUICK GUIDE

TARGET
• Transverse abdominals

TYPE
• Strengthening/stability

LEVEL
• Advanced

BENEFITS
• Stabilizes core
• Strengthens abdominals
• Strengthens lower back

NOT ADVISABLE IF YOU HAVE
• Severe neck pain
• Severe lower-back pain

DO IT RIGHT

DO
• Breathe easily and normally.
• Activate your abdominals so that you maintain neutral alignment.

AVOID
• Allowing your lower back to drop out of alignment.

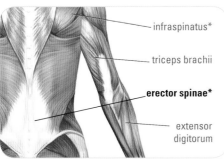

flexor digitorum*

extensor carpi radialis

flexor carpi radialis

BEST FOR

- rectus abdominis
- transversus abdominis
- rectus femoris
- iliacus
- iliopsoas
- latissimus dorsi
- obliquus externus
- obliquus internus
- pectoralis major
- teres major
- triceps brachii
- erector spinae

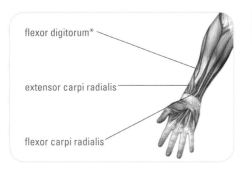

infraspinatus*

triceps brachii

erector spinae*

extensor digitorum

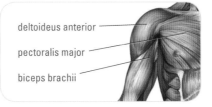

deltoideus anterior

pectoralis major

biceps brachii

ANNOTATION KEY
Bold text indicates active muscles
Gray text indicates stabilizing muscles
* indicates deep muscles

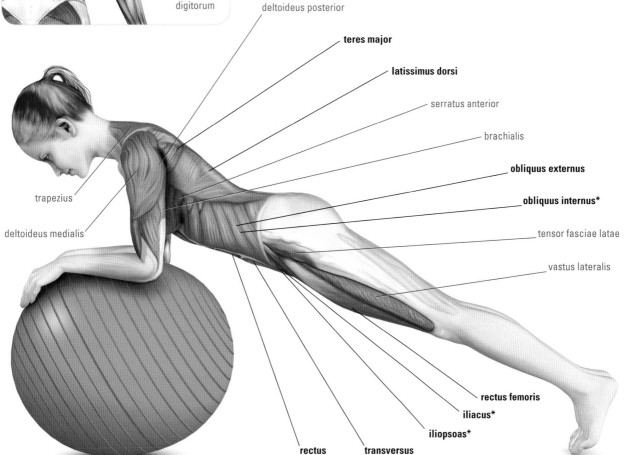

deltoideus posterior

teres major

latissimus dorsi

serratus anterior

brachialis

obliquus externus

obliquus internus*

tensor fasciae latae

vastus lateralis

trapezius

deltoideus medialis

rectus femoris

iliacus*

iliopsoas*

rectus abdominis

transversus abdominis

CROSSOVER CRUNCH

CORE

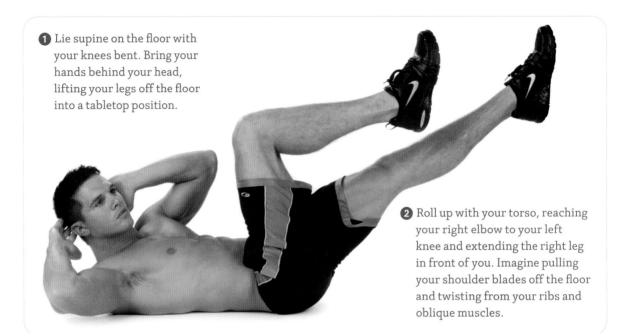

1 Lie supine on the floor with your knees bent. Bring your hands behind your head, lifting your legs off the floor into a tabletop position.

2 Roll up with your torso, reaching your right elbow to your left knee and extending the right leg in front of you. Imagine pulling your shoulder blades off the floor and twisting from your ribs and oblique muscles.

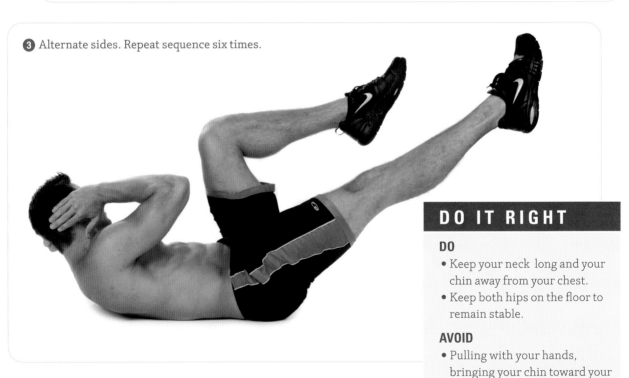

3 Alternate sides. Repeat sequence six times.

DO IT RIGHT

DO
- Keep your neck long and your chin away from your chest.
- Keep both hips on the floor to remain stable.

AVOID
- Pulling with your hands, bringing your chin toward your chest, or arching your back.
- Moving the active elbow faster than your shoulder.

MODIFICATION

Easier: Begin with both feet on the floor. Place the outside of one foot on top of your thigh near your knee. Reach your opposite elbow toward the knee of your raised leg. After six repetitions, repeat on the other side.

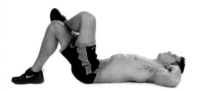

QUICK GUIDE

TARGET
- AbdominalsType
- StrengtheningLevel
- AdvancedBenefits
- Strengthens abdominals
- Stabilizes core

NOT ADVISABLE IF YOU HAVE
- Neck issues
- Lower-back pain

BEST FOR

- rectus abdominis
- transversus abdominis
- obliquus externus
- obliquus internus
- rectus femoris
- vastus medialis
- sartorius
- tensor fasciae latae

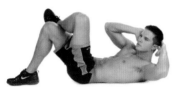

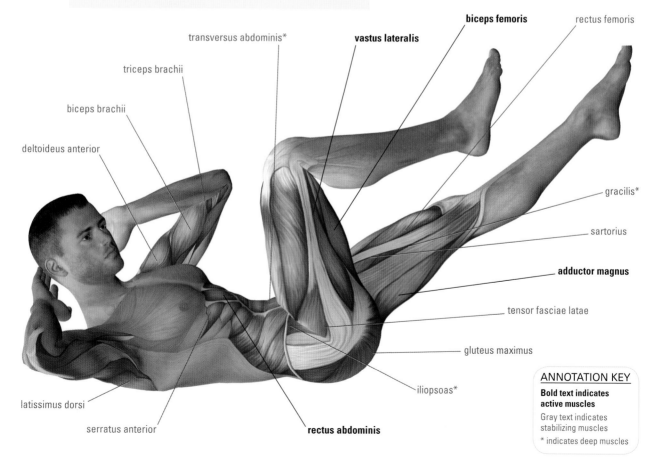

biceps femoris · rectus femoris · vastus lateralis · transversus abdominis* · triceps brachii · biceps brachii · deltoideus anterior · gracilis* · sartorius · adductor magnus · tensor fasciae latae · gluteus maximus · iliopsoas* · latissimus dorsi · serratus anterior · rectus abdominis

ANNOTATION KEY

Bold text indicates active muscles

Gray text indicates stabilizing muscles

* indicates deep muscles

THE TWIST

CORE

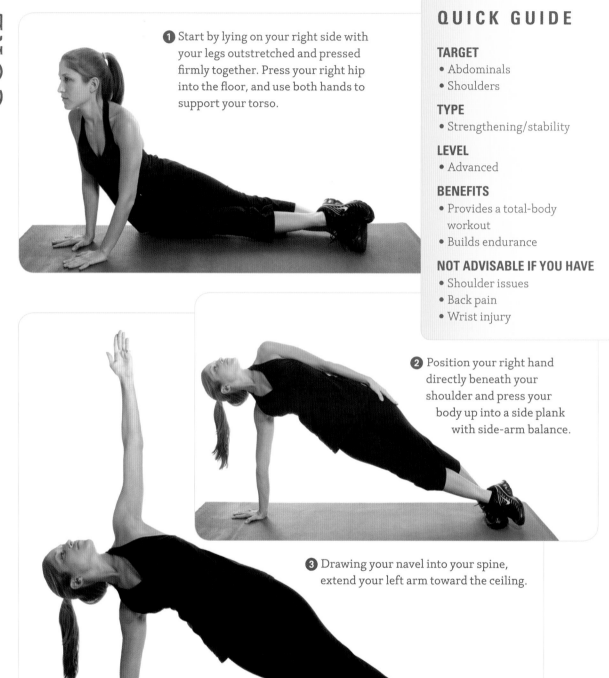

1 Start by lying on your right side with your legs outstretched and pressed firmly together. Press your right hip into the floor, and use both hands to support your torso.

2 Position your right hand directly beneath your shoulder and press your body up into a side plank with side-arm balance.

3 Drawing your navel into your spine, extend your left arm toward the ceiling.

QUICK GUIDE

TARGET
- Abdominals
- Shoulders

TYPE
- Strengthening/stability

LEVEL
- Advanced

BENEFITS
- Provides a total-body workout
- Builds endurance

NOT ADVISABLE IF YOU HAVE
- Shoulder issues
- Back pain
- Wrist injury

DO IT RIGHT

DO
- Keep your limbs elongated as much as possible.
- Keep your shoulders stable.
- Lift your hips up high to reduce the weight on your upper body.

AVOID
- Allowing your shoulder to sink into its socket.

BEST FOR

- latissimus dorsi
- rectus abdominis
- obliquus internus
- obliquus externus
- transversus abdominis
- adductor magnus
- adductor longus
- deltoideus

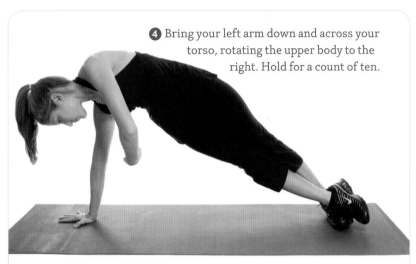

④ Bring your left arm down and across your torso, rotating the upper body to the right. Hold for a count of ten.

⑤ Return to the starting position, with your hip on the floor and both hands supporting your torso. Repeat sequence four to six times, and then switch sides.

ANNOTATION KEY
Bold text indicates active muscles
Gray text indicates stabilizing muscles
* indicates deep muscles

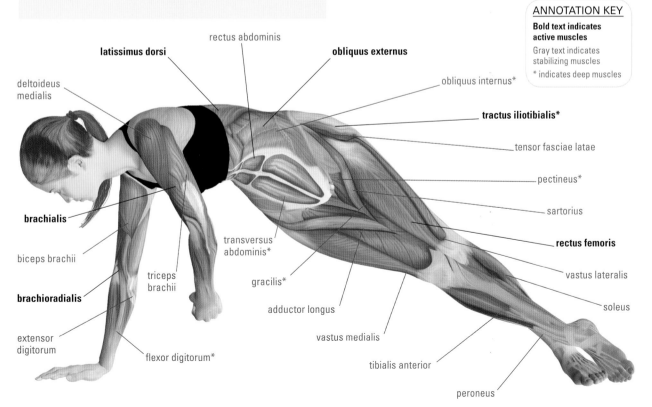

rectus abdominis

latissimus dorsi

obliquus externus

deltoideus medialis

obliquus internus*

tractus iliotibialis*

tensor fasciae latae

pectineus*

sartorius

brachialis

rectus femoris

biceps brachii

triceps brachii

transversus abdominis*

vastus lateralis

brachioradialis

gracilis*

soleus

adductor longus

extensor digitorum

vastus medialis

flexor digitorum*

tibialis anterior

peroneus

SIDE-BEND PLANK

CORE

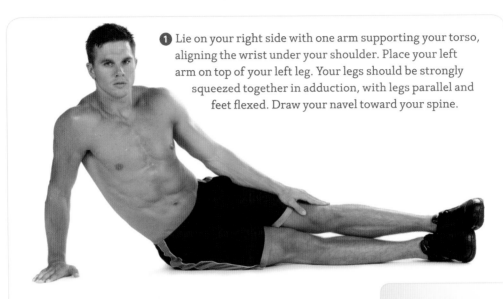

1 Lie on your right side with one arm supporting your torso, aligning the wrist under your shoulder. Place your left arm on top of your left leg. Your legs should be strongly squeezed together in adduction, with legs parallel and feet flexed. Draw your navel toward your spine.

BEST FOR

- rectus abdominis
- obliquus internus
- obliquus externus
- adductor magnus
- pectoralis major
- pectoralis minor
- triceps brachii
- gluteus medius

QUICK GUIDE

TARGET
- Abdominals
- Leg abductors and adductors
- Latissimus dorsi

TYPE
- Strengthening/stability

LEVEL
- Advanced

BENEFITS
- Stabilizes the spine in neutral position with the support of the shoulder girdle

NOT ADVISABLE IF YOU HAVE
- Rotator cuff injury
- Neck issues

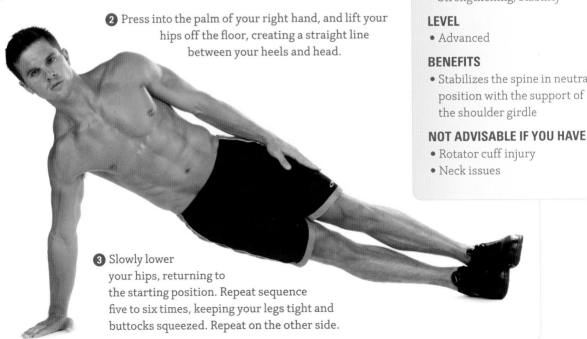

2 Press into the palm of your right hand, and lift your hips off the floor, creating a straight line between your heels and head.

3 Slowly lower your hips, returning to the starting position. Repeat sequence five to six times, keeping your legs tight and buttocks squeezed. Repeat on the other side.

MODIFICATION

Easier: Rather than supporting your torso with your arm straight, bend your elbow so that it is aligned below your shoulder.

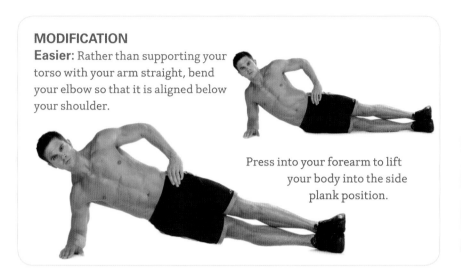

Press into your forearm to lift your body into the side plank position.

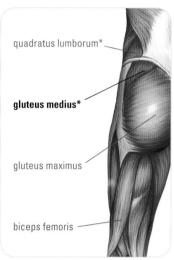

quadratus lumborum*

gluteus medius*

gluteus maximus

biceps femoris

ANNOTATION KEY

Bold text indicates active muscles
Gray text indicates stabilizing muscles
* indicates deep muscles

DO IT RIGHT

DO
• Lift your hips high to take some weight off your upper body.
• Elongate your limbs as much as possible.

AVOID
• Allowing your shoulders to sink into their sockets or lift toward your ears.

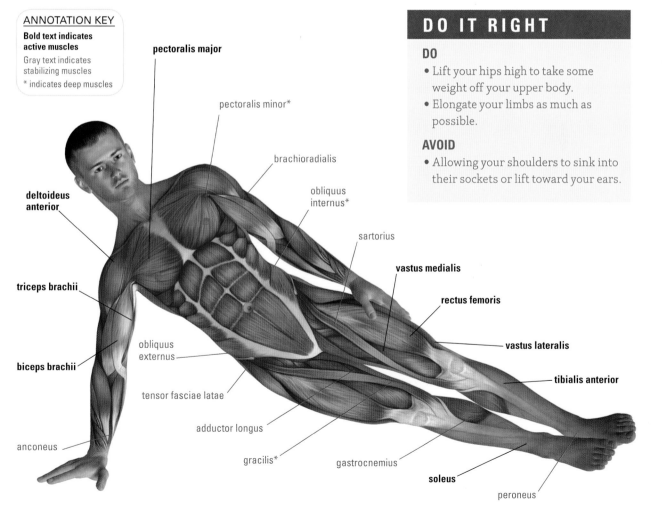

pectoralis major

pectoralis minor*

brachioradialis

obliquus internus*

sartorius

deltoideus anterior

vastus medialis

rectus femoris

triceps brachii

vastus lateralis

biceps brachii

obliquus externus

tibialis anterior

tensor fasciae latae

adductor longus

anconeus

gracilis*

gastrocnemius

soleus

peroneus

LUMBAR EXERCISES

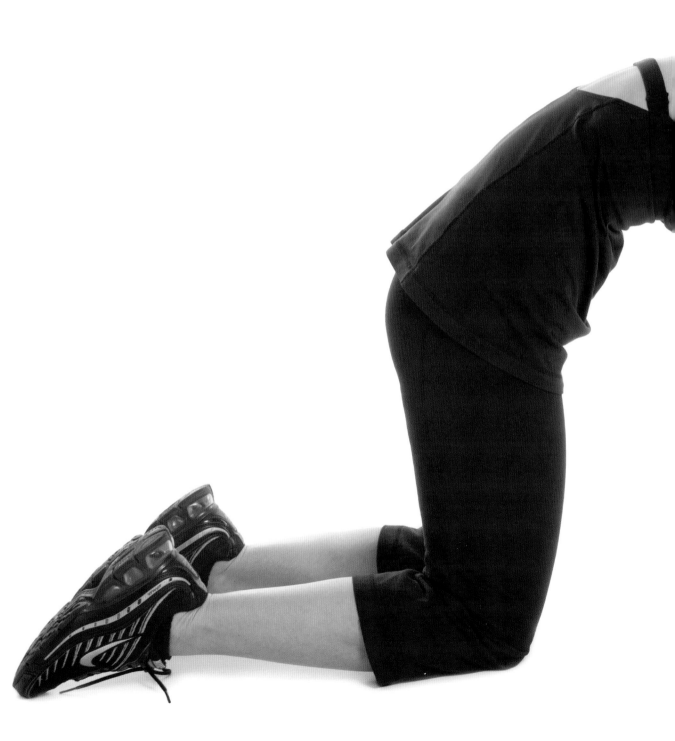

Lumbar, or lower-back, pain is one of the most common back complaints, with a vast majority of adults experiencing it at some point in their lives. For the many among us who have dealt with lumbar pain—and even for those lucky few who haven't—investing in an healthy back exercise regimen can increase strength and improve flexibility, which may help prevent future injury.

Sedentary lifestyles are a healthy back's enemy—without even simple exercise, the lumbar muscles can weaken easily. Weak back muscles not only leave you prey to injury, they also make it more difficult to recover if you are injured. An exercise plan that carefully targets the lower back will improve your physical conditioning, with the added bonus of helping you move efficiently and learn body awareness—both keys to lumbar injury prevention.

SUPINE PELVIC TILT

LUMBAR

QUICK GUIDE

TARGET
- Low back
- Abdominals

TYPE
- Stability

LEVEL
- Beginner

BENEFITS
- Improves posture
- Relieves lower-back pain

NOT ADVISABLE IF YOU HAVE
- Severe lower-back pain

1 Lie in a neutral position on your back with the knees bent and your feet flat on the floor. The natural curve of the lumbar spine should cause your low back to be slightly elevated from the floor.

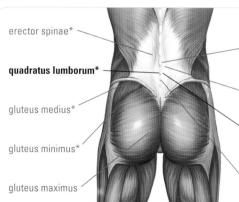

rectus abdominis
obliquus externus
transversus abdominis*
obliquus internus*
iliopsoas*
iliacus*

ANNOTATION KEY
Italic text indicates deep ligaments
Black text indicates joints
Bold text indicates active muscles
Gray text indicates stabilizing muscles
* indicates deep muscles

2 Exhale, and gently pull your belly button in toward your spine while rotating your hips posteriorly as you press your low back into the floor, taking the curve out of the low back.

3 Hold for two seconds, inhale, and return to your neutral position.

4 Repeat this movement ten times.

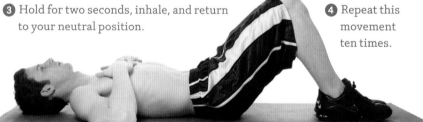

DO IT RIGHT

DO
- Use the 2-2-2 method: Take two seconds to get into position, hold for two seconds, and then release for two seconds. Advance to 2-5-2 as you progress.
- Tilt your pelvis toward your abdomen.

AVOID
- Lifting your buttocks off the floor.

BEST FOR

- rectus abdominis
- gluteus maximus
- gluteus medius
- gluteus minimus
- transversus abdominis
- ligamentum interspinalis
- ligamentum longitudinale posterius
- articulationes zygapophysiales
- ligamentum capsular facet

erector spinae*
quadratus lumborum*
gluteus medius*
gluteus minimus*
gluteus maximus

ligamentum longitudinale posterius

ligamentum interspinalis

articulationes zygapophysiales

ligamentum capsular facet

SEATED PELVIC TILT

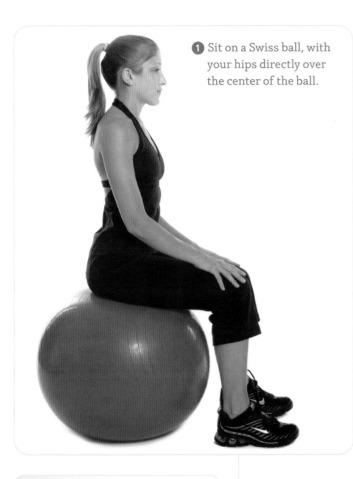

1 Sit on a Swiss ball, with your hips directly over the center of the ball.

BEST FOR

- rectus abdominis
- gluteus maximus
- gluteus medius
- gluteus minimus
- transversus abdominis

DO IT RIGHT

DO
- Make small movements—a correct pelvic tilt is a very subtle exercise.

AVOID
- Rounding your back too much— concentrate on moving your pelvis.

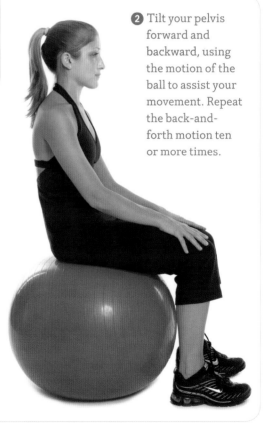

2 Tilt your pelvis forward and backward, using the motion of the ball to assist your movement. Repeat the back-and-forth motion ten or more times.

QUICK GUIDE

TARGET
- Back
- Abdominals
- Gluteal muscles

TYPE
- Stability

LEVEL
- Beginner

BENEFITS
- Improves posture
- Relieves lower-back pain

NOT ADVISABLE IF YOU HAVE
- Severe lower-back pain

TOE TOUCH

LUMBAR

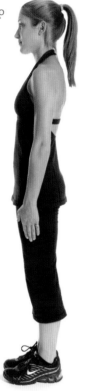

1 Stand up tall and exhale.

DO IT RIGHT

DO
- Stack your spine one vertebra at a time.
- Connect the stretch in your back with the stretch in your hamstrings.
- Make the stretch long and smooth.

AVOID
- Tensing your neck muscles.
- Bouncing as you try to reach your hands to your toes—reach down only as far as you can comfortably extend.

QUICK GUIDE

TARGET
- Spine

TYPE
- Flexibility

LEVEL
- Beginner

BENEFITS
- Stretches the spine and hamstrings
- Refines spinal stacking skills

NOT ADVISABLE IF YOU HAVE
- Lower-back pain that radiates down the leg

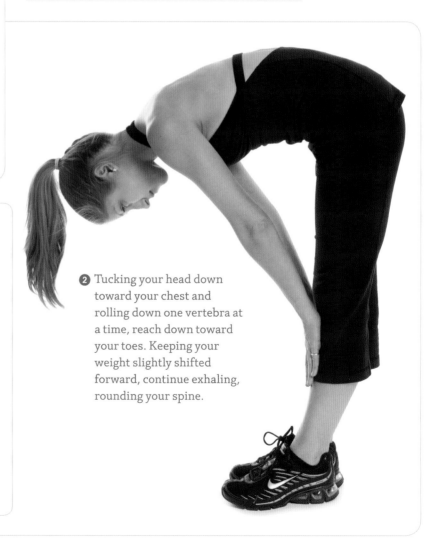

2 Tucking your head down toward your chest and rolling down one vertebra at a time, reach down toward your toes. Keeping your weight slightly shifted forward, continue exhaling, rounding your spine.

3 When you are completely folded over, inhale and begin uncurling your spine, stacking the spine from your hips up to your shoulders. Roll your shoulders back and stand up tall. Repeat three times.

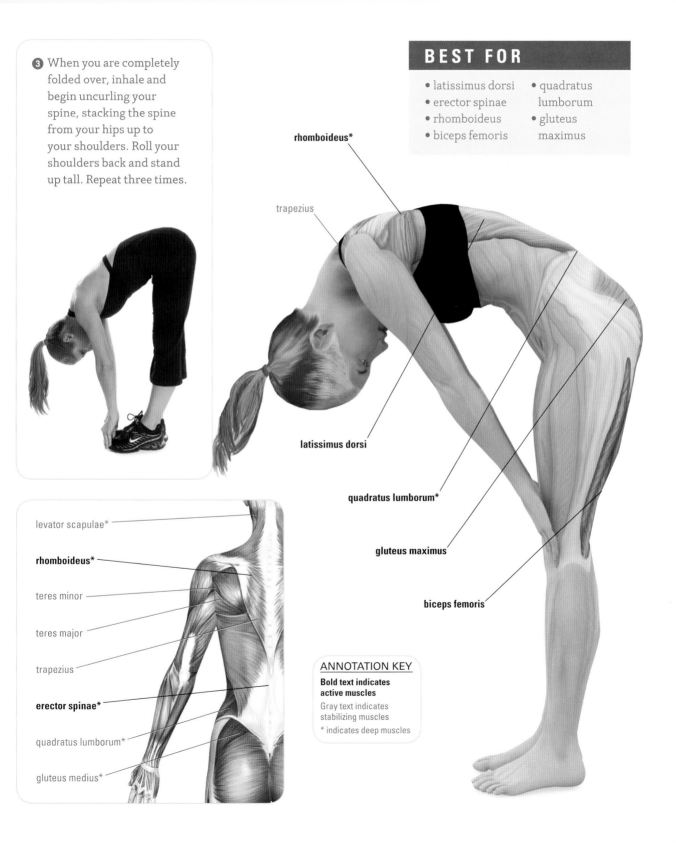

rhomboideus*

trapezius

latissimus dorsi

quadratus lumborum*

gluteus maximus

biceps femoris

levator scapulae*

rhomboideus*

teres minor

teres major

trapezius

erector spinae*

quadratus lumborum*

gluteus medius*

ANNOTATION KEY

Bold text indicates active muscles

Gray text indicates stabilizing muscles

* indicates deep muscles

KNEE-TO-CHEST HUG

LUMBAR

1 Lie supine on a mat with your legs together and arms outstretched.

2 Bend your right knee, and bring your foot to your body's midline while clasping your hands together to hold your knee. Hold the stretch for fifteen seconds.

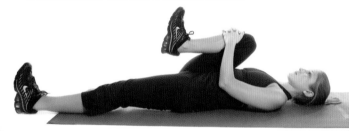

DO IT RIGHT

DO
• Keep your spine in neutral position.

AVOID
• Lifting your buttocks off the floor.

3 Return to the starting position.

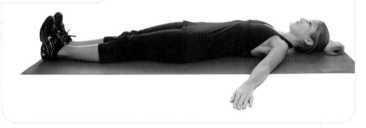

4 Again, clasping your hands together to hold your knee, bend your right knee, but this time rotate the right leg to the left, bringing the side of your leg against your chest.

5 Hold the stretch for fifteen seconds, and then return to the starting position. Repeat the entire sequence with the left leg bent.

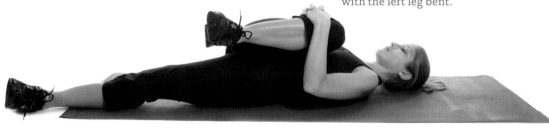

MODIFICATION
Similar difficulty: Follow step 1, and then draw both legs to your chest.

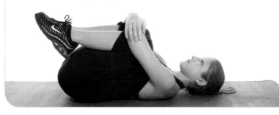

BEST FOR

- erector spinae
- latissimus dorsi
- gluteus maximus
- gluteus minimus
- piriformis
- gemellus superior
- gemellus inferior
- obturator externus
- obturator internus
- quadratus femoris

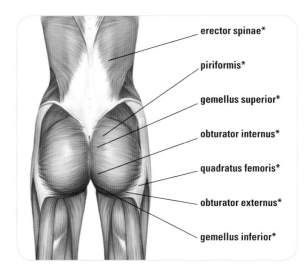

erector spinae*

piriformis*

gemellus superior*

obturator internus*

quadratus femoris*

obturator externus*

gemellus inferior*

QUICK GUIDE

TARGET
- Lower back
- Hips

TYPE
- Flexibility

LEVEL
- Beginner

BENEFITS
- Stretches lower back, hip extensors, and hip rotators

NOT ADVISABLE IF YOU HAVE
- Advanced degenerative joint disease

ANNOTATION KEY
Bold text indicates active muscles
Gray text indicates stabilizing muscles
* indicates deep muscles

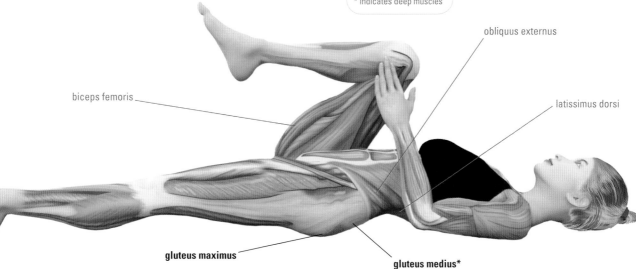

obliquus externus

biceps femoris

latissimus dorsi

gluteus maximus

gluteus medius*

SPINE STRETCH

LUMBAR

1 Lie on your back with your left leg straight and your right leg bent, placing your right foot on your left shin.

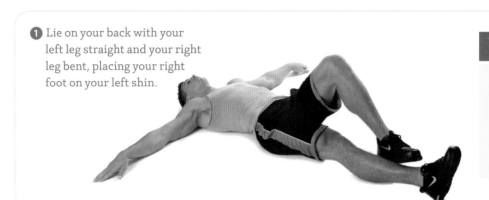

BEST FOR

- quadratus lumborum
- erector spinae
- vastus lateralis
- tractus iliotibialis
- tensor fasciae latae

DO IT RIGHT

DO
- Relax your lower back.

AVOID
- Allowing your shoulders to lift off the floor.

2 Keeping both shoulders on the floor, slowly bring your right leg across your body until you feel the stretch in the area between your lower back and hips. Stretch only as far as your shoulders will allow without one of them rising from the floor.

3 Hold for fifteen seconds, and repeat the sequence three times on each side.

QUICK GUIDE

TARGET
- Lower back

TYPE
- Flexibility

LEVEL
- Beginner

BENEFITS
- Increases lower-back flexibility

NOT ADVISABLE IF YOU HAVE
- Severe lower-back pain

ANNOTATION KEY

Bold text indicates active muscles

Gray text indicates stabilizing muscles

* indicates deep muscles

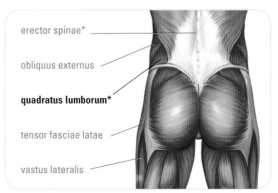

erector spinae*

obliquus externus

quadratus lumborum*

tensor fasciae latae

vastus lateralis

LOWER-BACK ROTATION

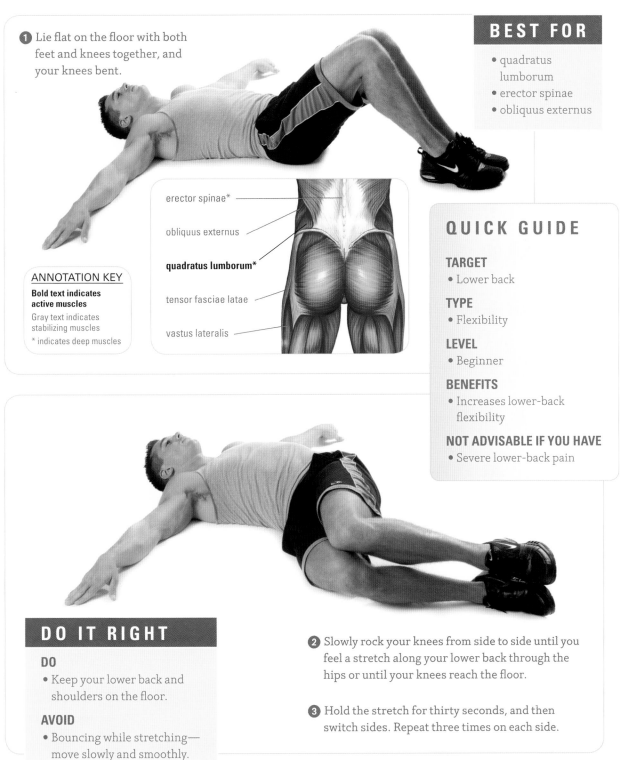

1 Lie flat on the floor with both feet and knees together, and your knees bent.

erector spinae*

obliquus externus

quadratus lumborum*

tensor fasciae latae

vastus lateralis

BEST FOR

- quadratus lumborum
- erector spinae
- obliquus externus

LUMBAR

QUICK GUIDE

TARGET
- Lower back

TYPE
- Flexibility

LEVEL
- Beginner

BENEFITS
- Increases lower-back flexibility

NOT ADVISABLE IF YOU HAVE
- Severe lower-back pain

DO IT RIGHT

DO
- Keep your lower back and shoulders on the floor.

AVOID
- Bouncing while stretching—move slowly and smoothly.

2 Slowly rock your knees from side to side until you feel a stretch along your lower back through the hips or until your knees reach the floor.

3 Hold the stretch for thirty seconds, and then switch sides. Repeat three times on each side.

CHILD'S POSE

LUMBAR

1 Kneel on a mat with your hips aligned over your knees. Bring your legs together so that your big toes are touching.

2 Sit back, resting your buttocks on your heels. Separate your knees about hip-width apart.

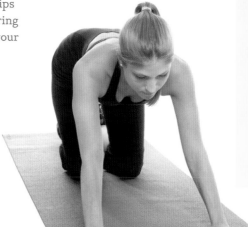

DO IT RIGHT

DO
• Round your back to create a dome shape.

AVOID
• Rushing the pose. It can take a few minutes to allow your body to deepen into the full stretch.
• Compressing the back of your neck.

3 Lower your chest onto your thighs as you extend your hands in front of your head, elongating your neck and spine as you stretch your tailbone toward the mat.

4 Place your forehead on the mat, and hold this position for thirty seconds to three minutes.

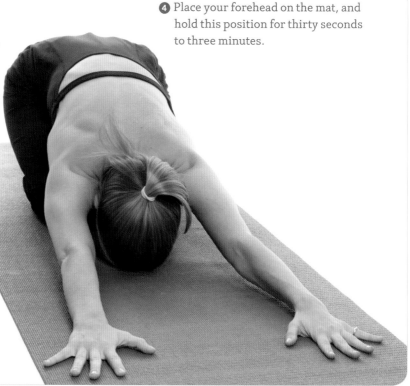

QUICK GUIDE

TARGET
• Lower back

TYPE
• Flexibility

LEVEL
• Beginner

BENEFITS
• Stretches and relaxes the back

NOT ADVISABLE IF YOU HAVE
• Knee injury

BEST FOR

- latissimus dorsi
- trapezius
- deltoideus anterior
- deltoideus posterior
- rhomboideus
- teres major
- serratus anterior
- gluteus maximus
- erector spinae
- quadratus lumborum

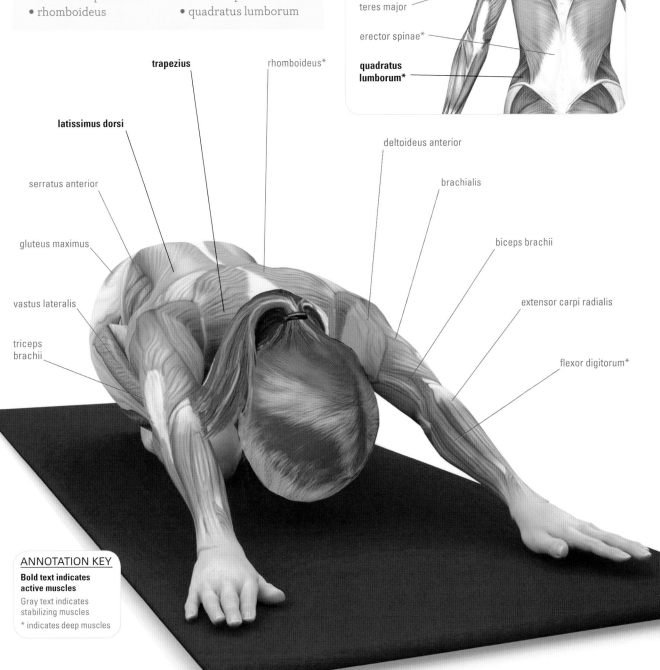

splenius*

deltoideus posterior

teres minor

teres major

erector spinae*

quadratus lumborum*

trapezius

rhomboideus*

latissimus dorsi

serratus anterior

deltoideus anterior

gluteus maximus

brachialis

vastus lateralis

biceps brachii

triceps brachii

extensor carpi radialis

flexor digitorum*

ANNOTATION KEY

Bold text indicates active muscles

Gray text indicates stabilizing muscles

* indicates deep muscles

CAT AND DOG STRETCH

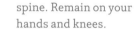

LUMBAR

① Begin on your hands and knees, with your wrists directly below your shoulders and your knees directly below your hips. Your fingertips should be facing forward, with your hands shoulder-width apart. Look down at the floor, keeping your head in a neutral position.

BEST FOR

- erector spinae
- multifidus spinae
- latissimus dorsi
- trapezius
- deltoideus posterior
- deltoideus anterior
- deltoideus medialis
- rectus abdominis
- transversus abdominis
- ligamentum longitudinale posterius
- articulationes zygapophysiales

② Exhale, and round your spine up toward the ceiling, dropping your head. Draw your belly button in toward your spine. Keep your hips lifted and your shoulders in the same position. This is the Cat pose.

③ Inhale, and uncurl your spine. Remain on your hands and knees.

④ With your next inhalation, arch your spine, lifting your chest forward and your tailbone toward the ceiling. Look forward. This is the Dog pose.

⑤ Exhale, and return to a neutral position on your hands and knees.

⑥ Repeat the entire sequence ten to twenty times.

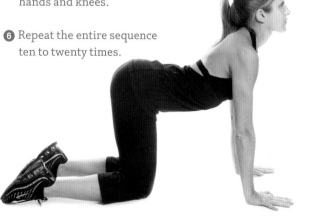

DO IT RIGHT

DO
- Draw your shoulders away from your neck.

AVOID
- Arching primarily in your lower back.
- Tucking your chin to your chest in the Cat pose.
- Jutting your rib cage out in the Dog pose.

QUICK GUIDE

TARGET
- Lower- and middle-back extensors
- Abdominals
- Obliques

TYPE
- Flexibility

LEVEL
- Beginner

BENEFITS
- Stretches shoulders, chest, abdominals, neck, and spine
- Improves range of motion

NOT ADVISABLE IF YOU HAVE
- Knee injury

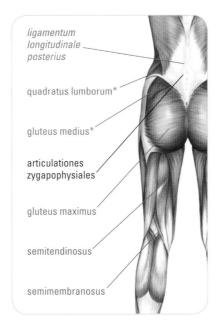

ligamentum longitudinale posterius

quadratus lumborum*

gluteus medius*

articulationes zygapophysiales

gluteus maximus

semitendinosus

semimembranosus

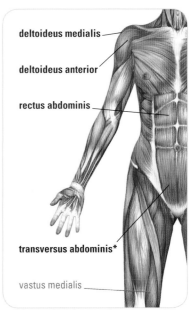

deltoideus medialis

deltoideus anterior

rectus abdominis

transversus abdominis*

vastus medialis

ANNOTATION KEY
Italic text indicates deep ligaments
Black text indicates joints
Bold text indicates active muscles
Gray text indicates stabilizing muscles
* indicates deep muscles

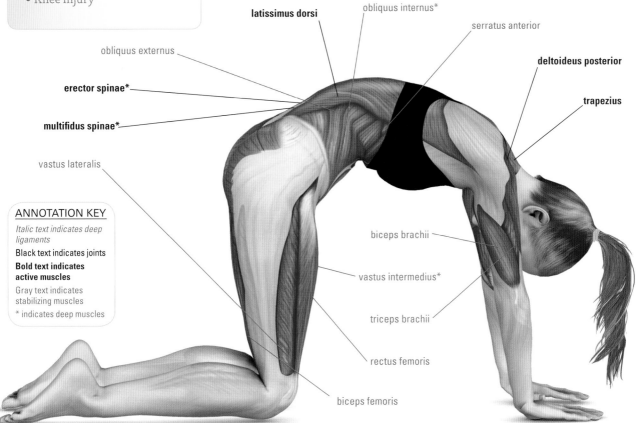

latissimus dorsi

obliquus internus*

serratus anterior

obliquus externus

erector spinae*

multifidus spinae*

vastus lateralis

deltoideus posterior

trapezius

biceps brachii

vastus intermedius*

triceps brachii

rectus femoris

biceps femoris

HIP CIRCLES

LUMBAR

1 Sit on a Swiss ball with your feet together and your hands on your hips.

QUICK GUIDE

TARGET
• Lower back
• Hips
• Abdominals

TYPE
• Flexibility/stability

LEVEL
• Intermediate

BENEFITS
• Stabilizes core
• Stretches lower back

NOT ADVISABLE IF YOU HAVE
• Severe lower-back pain

2 Tighten your abdominal muscles, and use your pelvis to rotate the ball slowly to the right in small counterclockwise circles.

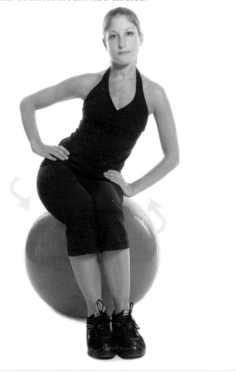

3 Return to the starting position, and repeat on the other side.

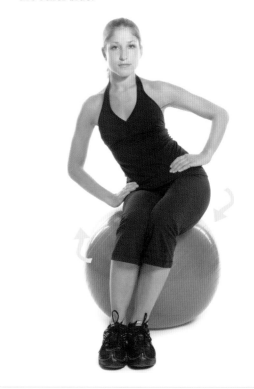

BEST FOR

- erector spinae
- multifidus spinae
- transversus abdominis
- obliquus externus
- quadratus lumborum
- infraspinatus
- gluteus medius
- iliopsoas
- iliacus

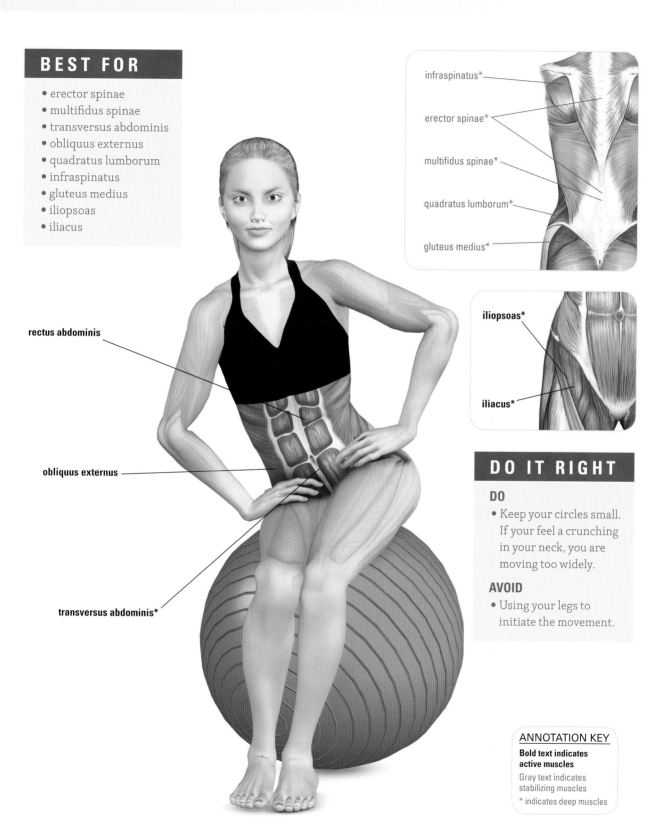

infraspinatus*

erector spinae*

multifidus spinae*

quadratus lumborum*

gluteus medius*

iliopsoas*

iliacus*

rectus abdominis

obliquus externus

transversus abdominis*

DO IT RIGHT

DO
- Keep your circles small. If your feel a crunching in your neck, you are moving too widely.

AVOID
- Using your legs to initiate the movement.

ANNOTATION KEY
Bold text indicates active muscles
Gray text indicates stabilizing muscles
* indicates deep muscles

SWIMMING

LUMBAR

1. Lie prone on the floor with your legs hip-width apart. Stretch your arms upward beside your ears on the floor. Engage your pelvic floor, and draw your belly button in toward your spine.

2. Extend through your upper back as you lift your left arm and right leg simultaneously. Lift your head and shoulders off the floor.

3. Lower your arm and leg to the starting position, maintaining a stretch in your limbs throughout.

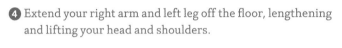

4. Extend your right arm and left leg off the floor, lengthening and lifting your head and shoulders.

5. Elongate your limbs as you return to the starting position. Repeat six to eight times.

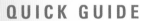

QUICK GUIDE

TARGET
- Spinal extensors
- Hip extensors

TYPE
- Stability/strengthening

LEVEL
- Intermediate

BENEFITS
- Strengthens hip and spine extensors
- Challenges stabilization of the spine against rotation

NOT ADVISABLE IF YOU HAVE
- Severe lower-back pain
- Extreme curvature of the upper spine
- Curvature of the lower spine

BEST FOR

- gluteus maximus
- trapezius
- biceps femoris
- erector spinae
- quadratus lumborum
- rhomboideus
- latissimus dorsi

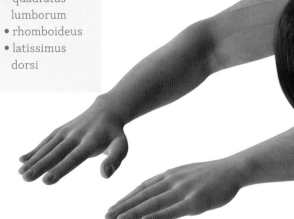

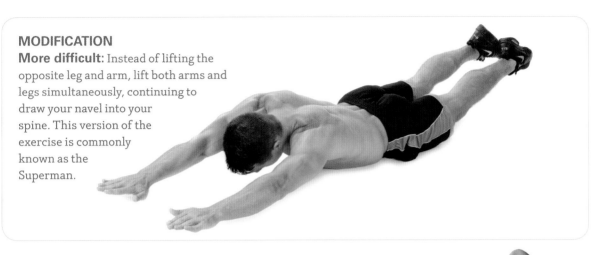

MODIFICATION

More difficult: Instead of lifting the opposite leg and arm, lift both arms and legs simultaneously, continuing to draw your navel into your spine. This version of the exercise is commonly known as the Superman.

ANNOTATION KEY

Bold text indicates active muscles

Gray text indicates stabilizing muscles

* indicates deep muscles

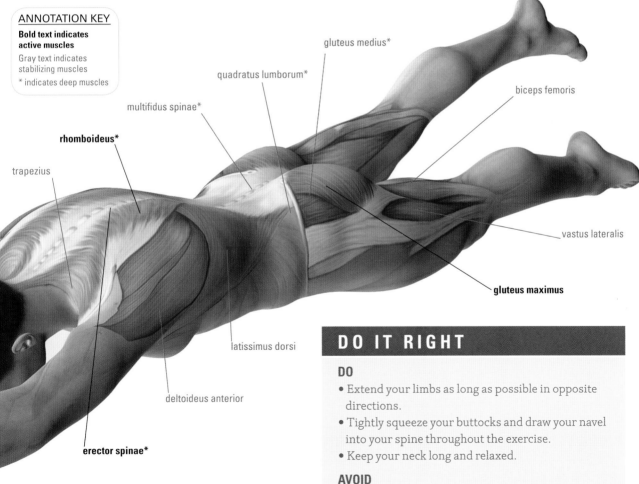

gluteus medius*

quadratus lumborum*

biceps femoris

multifidus spinae*

rhomboideus*

trapezius

vastus lateralis

gluteus maximus

latissimus dorsi

deltoideus anterior

erector spinae*

DO IT RIGHT

DO

• Extend your limbs as long as possible in opposite directions.
• Tightly squeeze your buttocks and draw your navel into your spine throughout the exercise.
• Keep your neck long and relaxed.

AVOID

• Allowing your shoulders to lift toward your ears.

BRIDGE

LUMBAR

❶ Lie supine on the floor. Bend your knees and draw your heels close to your buttocks. Place your hands flat on the floor by your sides.

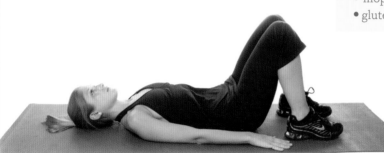

BEST FOR

- erector spinae
- iliopsoas
- gluteus maximus
- gluteus medius
- sartorius
- rectus femoris

QUICK GUIDE

TARGET
- Lower back
- Quadriceps
- Gluteal muscles
- Chest

TYPE
- Strengthening

LEVEL
- Intermediate

BENEFITS
- Strengthens thighs and buttocks
- Stretches chest and spine

NOT ADVISABLE IF YOU HAVE
- Shoulder injury
- Back injury
- Neck issues

❷ Exhale, and press down through your feet to lift your buttocks off the floor. With your feet and thighs parallel, push your arms into the floor while extending through your fingertips.

❸ Lengthen your neck away from your shoulders. Lift your hips higher so that your torso rises from the floor.

❹ Hold for thirty seconds to one minute. Exhale as you release your spine onto the floor, one vertebra at a time. Repeat at least one more time.

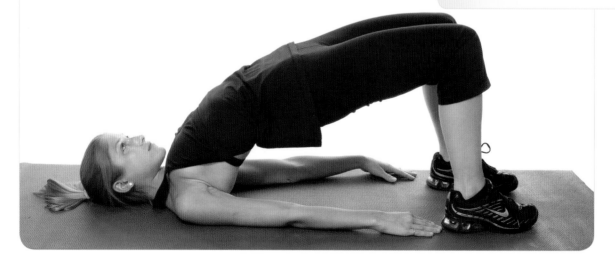

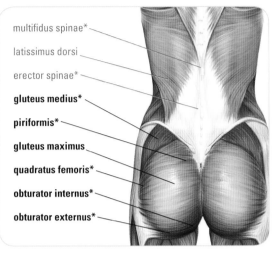

multifidus spinae*
latissimus dorsi
erector spinae*
gluteus medius*
piriformis*
gluteus maximus
quadratus femoris*
obturator internus*
obturator externus*

ANNOTATION KEY

Bold text indicates active muscles
Gray text indicates stabilizing muscles
* indicates deep muscles

DO IT RIGHT

DO
- Roll your shoulders under once your hips are raised.
- Keep your knees over your heels.
- Tighten your buttocks and your thighs.

AVOID
- Tucking your chin in toward your chest.
- Using your buttocks more than your hamstrings to lift your hips.

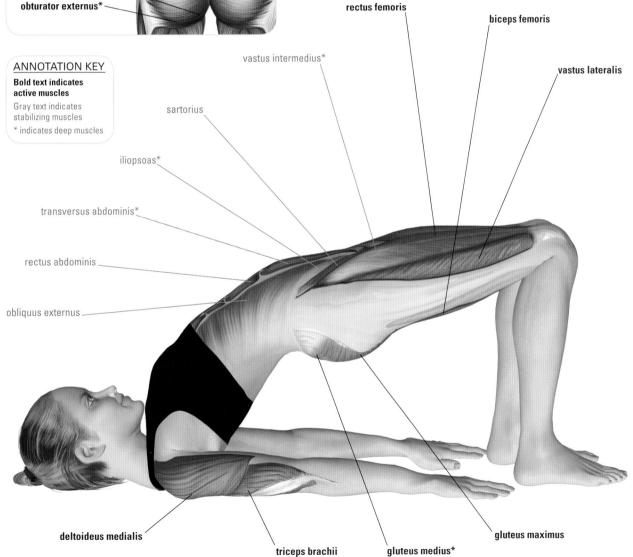

rectus femoris

biceps femoris

vastus lateralis

vastus intermedius*

sartorius

iliopsoas*

transversus abdominis*

rectus abdominis

obliquus externus

deltoideus medialis

triceps brachii

gluteus medius*

gluteus maximus

BRIDGE WITH LEG LIFT

LUMBAR

1 Lie supine on the floor. Bend your knees and draw your heels close to your buttocks. Place your hands flat on the floor by your sides.

2 Exhale, and press down through your feet to lift your buttocks off the floor. With your feet and thighs parallel, push your arms into the floor while extending through your fingertips.

3 Lengthen your neck away from your shoulders. Lift your hips higher so that your torso rises from the floor.

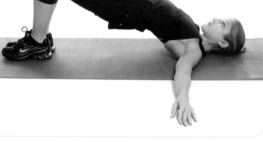

4 Straighten your right leg so that it is fully extended, forming a straight line from hip to toe.

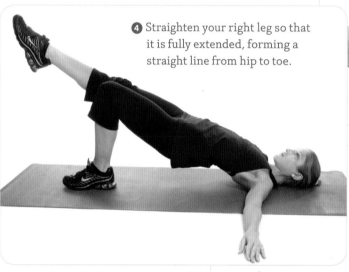

5 Hold for thirty seconds to one minute.

6 Return to the bridge position, and switch legs. Repeat the entire sequence at least one more time.

DO IT RIGHT

DO
- Your body should form a straight line from sternum to extended toe.
- The top of your sternum should be lifted forward.

AVOID
- Overextending your lumbar spine.

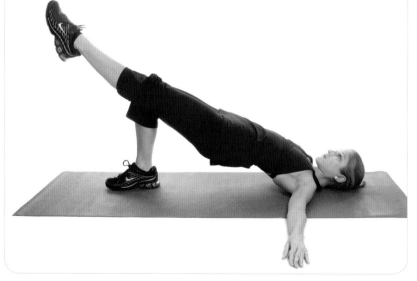

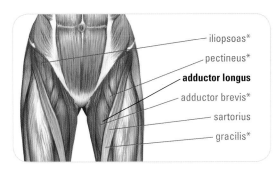

- iliopsoas*
- pectineus*
- **adductor longus**
- adductor brevis*
- sartorius
- gracilis*

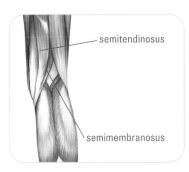

- semitendinosus
- semimembranosus

BEST FOR

- gluteus maximus
- gluteus medius
- erector spinae
- rectus femoris
- transversus abdominis

MODIFICATION

More difficult: Follow steps 1 through 5, and then draw your hands together, keeping your arms straight. Hold for thirty seconds to one minute. Return to bridge position, and switch legs. Repeat entire sequence at least one more time.

QUICK GUIDE

TARGET
- Lower back
- Quadriceps
- Gluteal muscles
- Abdominals

TYPE
- Strengthening/balance

LEVEL
- Advanced

BENEFITS
- Strengthens thighs and buttocks
- Stretches chest and spine

NOT ADVISABLE IF YOU HAVE
- Shoulder injury
- Back injury
- Neck issues

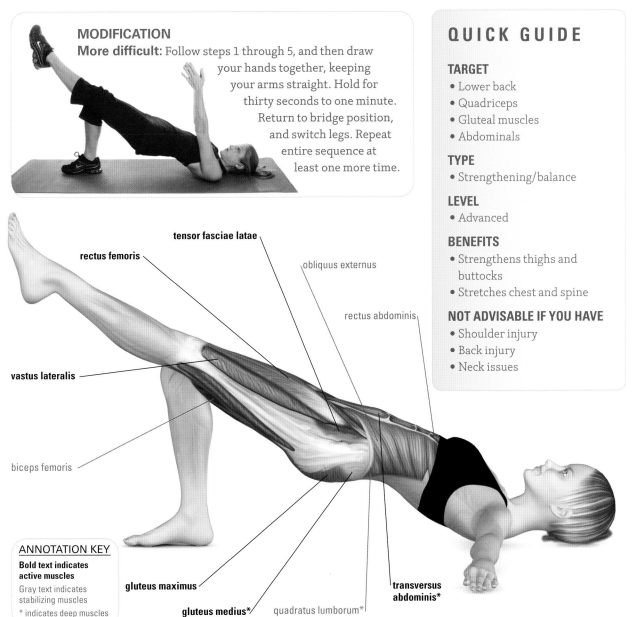

- **tensor fasciae latae**
- **rectus femoris**
- obliquus externus
- rectus abdominis
- **vastus lateralis**
- biceps femoris
- **gluteus maximus**
- **gluteus medius***
- quadratus lumborum*
- **transversus abdominis***

ANNOTATION KEY

Bold text indicates active muscles

Gray text indicates stabilizing muscles

* indicates deep muscles

LOWER-BODY EXERCISES

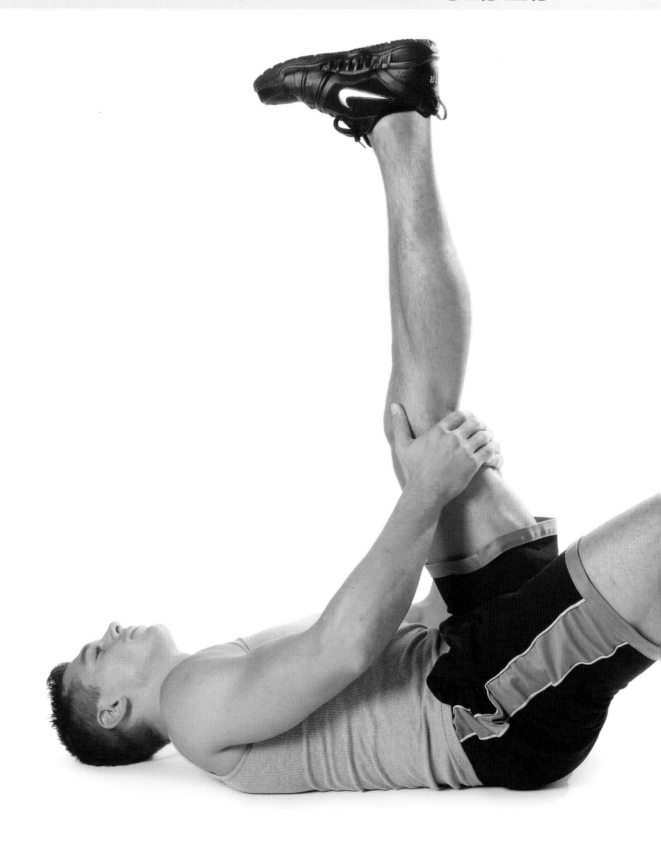

Although you might not think about a hamstring or quadriceps stretch when you are devising an exercise regimen that targets the back, if your goal is developing a supple, healthy back, adding several lower-body stretches, along with a few strengthening and stability exercises, is ideal. A conditioned lower body and strong legs can take stress off the lower back—a real bonus for those of us who spend long days on our feet. Along with the following stretches and exercises, try to incorporate walking into your fitness plan, especially if you have already suffered from back pain. Walking briskly for about twenty to thirty minutes not only benefits your legs, it can also boost your heart rate and lung function.

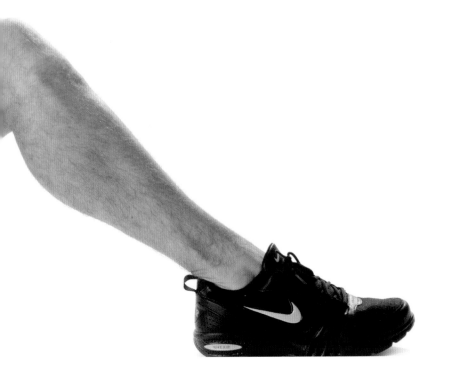

QUADRICEPS STRETCH

LOWER BODY

1 Stand with your feet together and your arms hanging loosely at your sides.

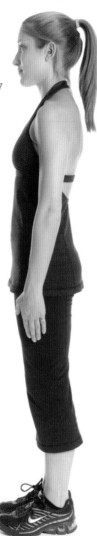

2 Balancing on your right leg, bend your left leg behind you, and grasp your foot with your left hand.

3 While pushing your hips forward, pull your heel toward your buttocks until you feel a stretch in the front of your thigh. Keep both knees together and aligned.

4 Hold for fifteen seconds. Repeat the sequence three times on each leg.

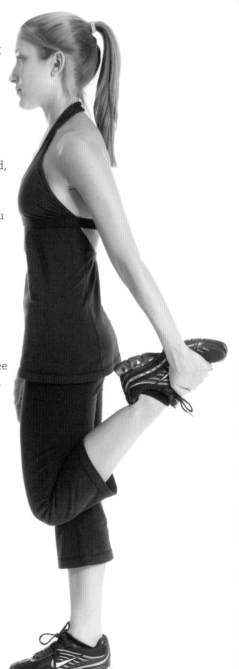

DO IT RIGHT

DO
- Keep both knees pressed together.

AVOID
- Leaning forward with your chest.

QUICK GUIDE

TARGET
- Quadriceps
- Hip flexors
- Knee extensors
- Anterior hip joint capsule

TYPE
- Flexibility

LEVEL
- Beginner

BENEFITS
- Relieves stiffness caused by sitting too long
- Increases the flexibility of the thighs, hips, and knees

NOT ADVISABLE IF YOU HAVE
- Knee injury
- Hip injury

BEST FOR

- rectus femoris
- vastus lateralis
- vastus medialis
- vastus intermedius

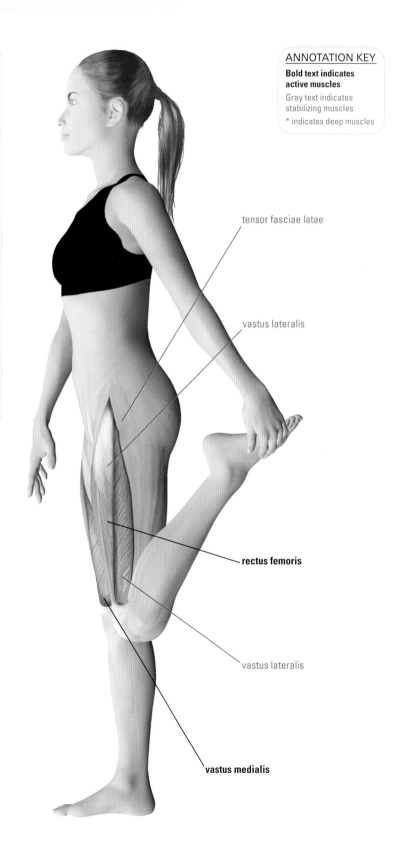

ANNOTATION KEY
Bold text indicates active muscles
Gray text indicates stabilizing muscles
* indicates deep muscles

tensor fasciae latae

vastus lateralis

rectus femoris

vastus lateralis

vastus medialis

ILIOTIBIAL BAND STRETCH

LOWER BODY

1 Standing, cross your left leg in front of your right.

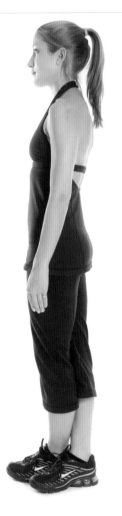

2 Bend at the waist while keeping both knees straight, and reach your hands toward the floor.

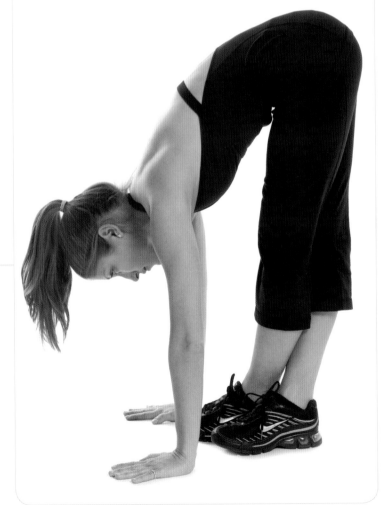

DO IT RIGHT

DO
- Keep your knees extended.
- Look for a long, smooth stretch.

AVOID
- Bouncing as you try to reach your hands to the floor—reach down only as far as you can comfortably extend.

3 Hold for fifteen seconds. Repeat the sequence three times on each leg.

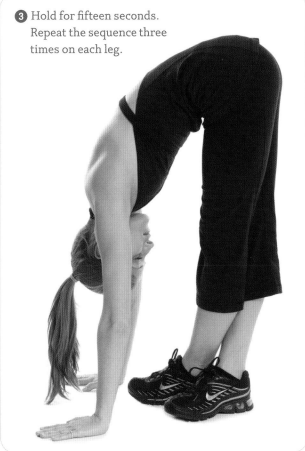

QUICK GUIDE

TARGET
• Iliotibial band

TYPE
• Flexibility

LEVEL
• Beginner

BENEFITS
• Stabilizes core
• Strengthens abdominals

NOT ADVISABLE IF YOU HAVE
• Neck issues
• Lower-back pain

ANNOTATION KEY
**Bold text indicates
active muscles**
Gray text indicates
stabilizing muscles
* indicates deep muscles

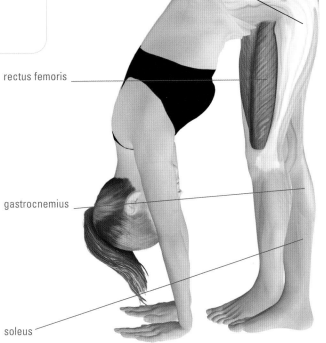

tractus iliotibialis

rectus femoris

gastrocnemius

soleus

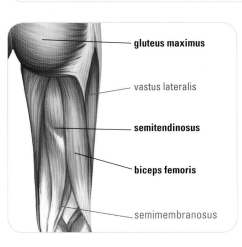

gluteus maximus

vastus lateralis

semitendinosus

biceps femoris

semimembranosus

HAMSTRING STRETCH I

LOWER BODY

1. Stand with your feet together and your arms hanging at your sides.

2. Extend your left leg so that your left heel is positioned about one foot beyond your right toes.

3. Keeping your left knee straight, bend your right knee while leaning forward to reach your left hand to the toes of your left foot.

4. Hold the stretch for five seconds, and then return to the starting position.

5. Repeat five times on each side.

BEST FOR

- semitendinosus
- semimembranosus
- biceps femoris
- gluteus maximus
- erector spinae
- gastrocnemius

QUICK GUIDE

TARGET
- Hamstrings
- Knee flexors

TYPE
- Flexibility

LEVEL
- Beginner

BENEFITS
- Relieves stiffness caused by sitting too long
- Increases the flexibility of the thighs, hips, and knees

NOT ADVISABLE IF YOU HAVE
- Knee pain
- Low-back pain

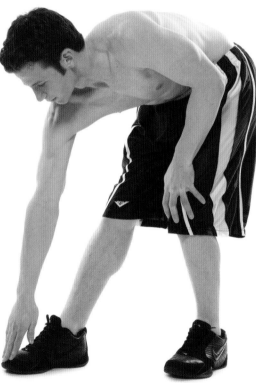

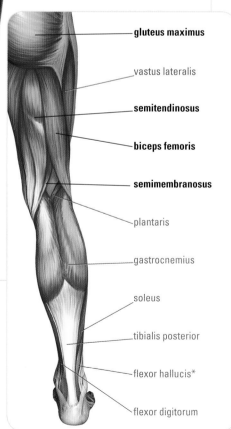

gluteus maximus

vastus lateralis

semitendinosus

biceps femoris

semimembranosus

plantaris

gastrocnemius

soleus

tibialis posterior

flexor hallucis*

flexor digitorum

DO IT RIGHT

DO
- Bend forward from the hips.

AVOID
- Bending the extended knee.

ANNOTATION KEY
Bold text indicates active muscles
Gray text indicates stabilizing muscles
* indicates deep muscles

HAMSTRING STRETCH II

LOWER BODY

❶ Lie on your back with both knees bent and your feet flat on the floor.

❷ Grasp your right leg behind the knee, and draw your knee in toward your chest.

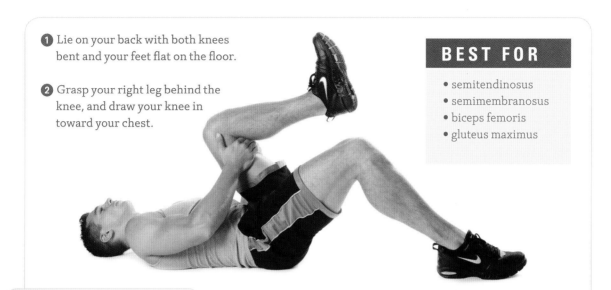

BEST FOR

- semitendinosus
- semimembranosus
- biceps femoris
- gluteus maximus

QUICK GUIDE

TARGET
- Hamstrings

TYPE
- Flexibility

LEVEL
- Beginner

BENEFITS
- Relieves stiffness caused by sitting too long
- Increases the flexibility of the thighs, hips, and knees

NOT ADVISABLE IF YOU HAVE
- Knee pain

❸ Keeping your knee pulled into your chest, flex your toes and contract your quadriceps, so that you begin to straighten your leg.

❹ Release your leg into the stretch, and pull it closer toward your chest. Repeat ten times on each leg.

DO IT RIGHT

DO
- Pull your knee toward your chest throughout the movement.
- Relax your neck and shoulders.
- Flex your toes.

AVOID
- Rounding your shoulders and lifting your head.
- Rolling your stabilizing leg out of neutral position.

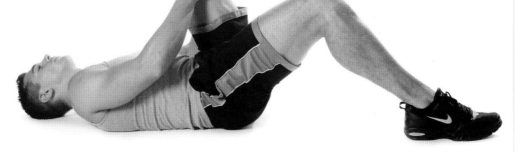

FORWARD LUNGE

LOWER BODY

① Stand with your feet together and your arms hanging at your sides.

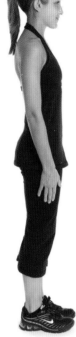

DO IT RIGHT

DO
• Maintain proper position of your shoulders and your whole upper body to lengthen your spine.

AVOID
• Dropping your back-extended knee to the floor.

② Exhale, and carefully step back with your right leg, keeping it in line with your hips as you step back. The ball of your left foot should be in contact with the floor as you do the motion.

③ Slowly slide your right foot farther back while bending your left knee, stacking it directly above your ankle.

④ Position your palms or fingers on the floor on either side of your left leg, and slowly press your palms or fingers against the floor to enhance the placement of your upper body and your head.

⑤ Lift your head and gaze straight forward while leaning your upper body forward and carefully rolling your shoulders down and backward.

⑥ Press the ball of your right foot gradually on the floor, contract your thigh muscles, and press up to maintain your left leg in a straight position.

⑦ Hold for five seconds. Slowly return to the starting position, and then repeat on the other side.

QUICK GUIDE

TARGET
• Quadriceps
• Hamstrings
• Calf muscles

TYPE
• Flexibility/strengthening

LEVEL
• Intermediate

BENEFITS
• Strengthens legs and arms
• Stretches groins

NOT ADVISABLE IF YOU HAVE
• Arm injury
• Shoulder injury
• Hip injury
• High or low blood pressure

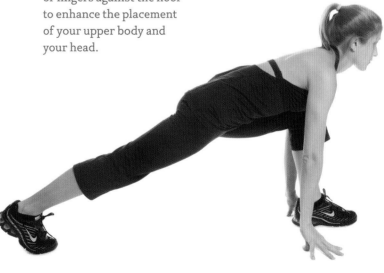

MODIFICATION

More difficult: Follow steps 1 through 3, using your right leg as the forward leg. Then position the palm of your left hand on the floor. Place your right hand behind your head, and slowly try to touch your elbow to the inside of your right ankle. Return to the starting position, and then repeat on the other side.

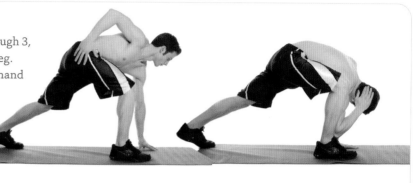

BEST FOR

- biceps femoris
- adductor longus
- adductor magnus
- gastrocnemius
- tibialis posterior
- iliopsoas
- biceps femoris
- rectus femoris

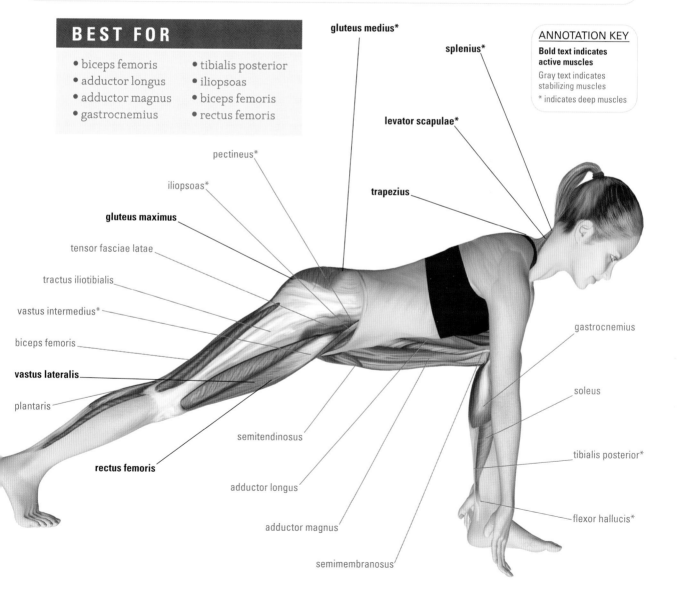

gluteus medius*

splenius*

levator scapulae*

trapezius

pectineus*

iliopsoas*

gluteus maximus

tensor fasciae latae

tractus iliotibialis

vastus intermedius*

biceps femoris

vastus lateralis

plantaris

rectus femoris

semitendinosus

adductor longus

adductor magnus

semimembranosus

gastrocnemius

soleus

tibialis posterior*

flexor hallucis*

HIP FLEXOR STRETCH

LOWER BODY

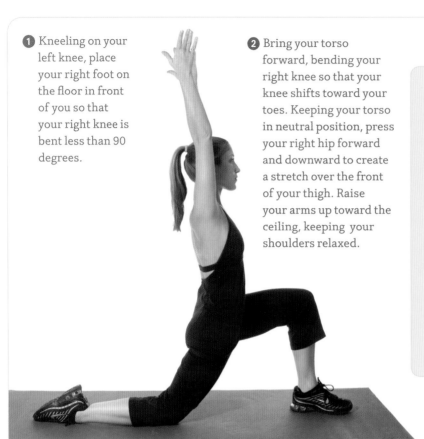

1 Kneeling on your left knee, place your right foot on the floor in front of you so that your right knee is bent less than 90 degrees.

2 Bring your torso forward, bending your right knee so that your knee shifts toward your toes. Keeping your torso in neutral position, press your right hip forward and downward to create a stretch over the front of your thigh. Raise your arms up toward the ceiling, keeping your shoulders relaxed.

QUICK GUIDE

TARGET
• Quadriceps
• Hamstrings

TYPE
• Flexibility

LEVEL
• Intermediate

BENEFITS
• Stretches hip flexors and extensors

NOT ADVISABLE IF YOU HAVE
• Severe neck pain
• Severe lower-back pain

DO IT RIGHT

DO
• Keep your shoulders and neck relaxed.
• Move your entire body as one unit as you go into the stretch.

AVOID
• Extending your front knee too far over the planted foot.
• Rotating your hips.
• Shifting the knee of the back leg outward.

3 Bring your arms down and move your hips backward. Straighten your right leg, and bring your torso forward. Place your hands on either side of your straight leg for support.

4 Hold for ten seconds, and repeat the forward and backward movement five times on each leg.

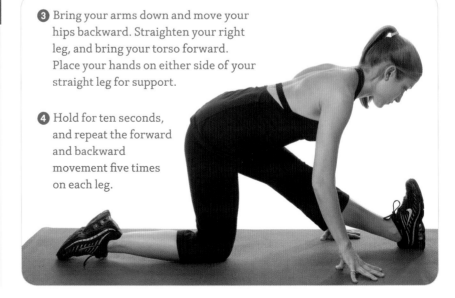

MODIFICATION

More difficult: During the backward movement, raise your back knee off the floor and straighten your back leg. Keep your hands on the floor.

BEST FOR

- iliacus
- iliopsoas
- biceps femoris
- rectus femoris

iliopsoas*
iliacus*
tensor fasciae latae
pectineus*
adductor longus
rectus femoris
gracilis*

ANNOTATION KEY
Bold text indicates active muscles
Gray text indicates stabilizing muscles
* indicates deep muscles

obliquus externus

latissimus dorsi

biceps femoris

vastus lateralis

semimembranosus

gastrocnemius

rectus abdominis

adductor magnus

vastus intermedius*

vastus medialis

semitendinosus

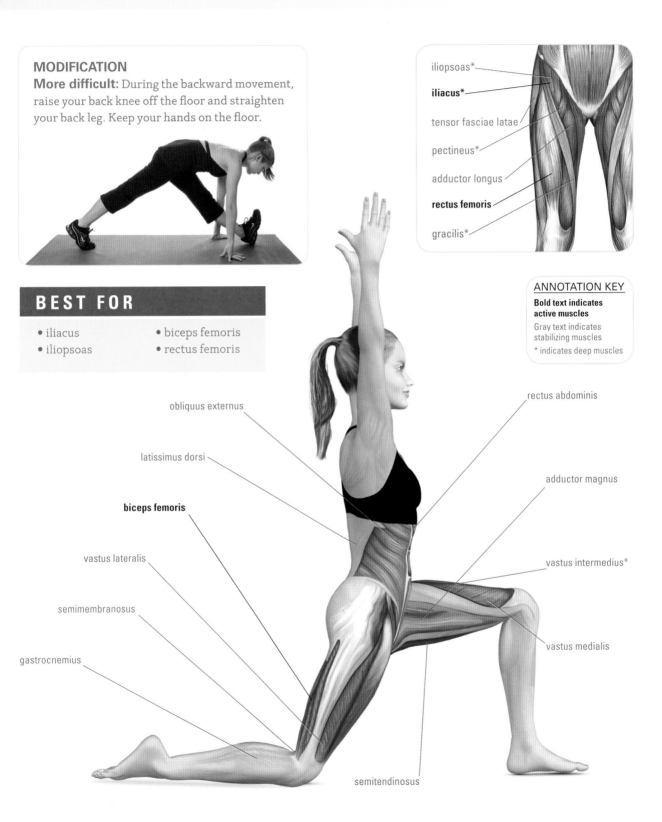

HIP STRETCH

LOWER BODY

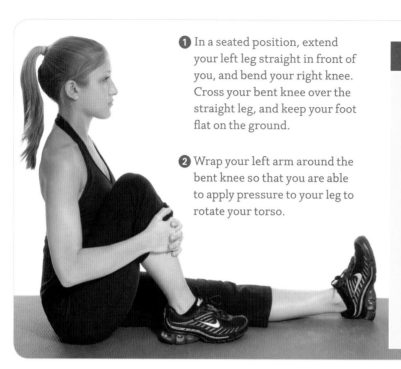

❶ In a seated position, extend your left leg straight in front of you, and bend your right knee. Cross your bent knee over the straight leg, and keep your foot flat on the ground.

❷ Wrap your left arm around the bent knee so that you are able to apply pressure to your leg to rotate your torso.

DO IT RIGHT

DO
• Keep your neck and shoulders relaxed.
• Apply even pressure to your leg with your active hand.
• Keep your torso upright as you pull your knee and torso together.

AVOID
• Rounding your torso.
• Lifting the foot of your bent leg off the floor.
• Straining your neck as you rotate.

BEST FOR

• adductor longus
• iliopsoas
• rhomboideus
• sternocleidomastoideus
• latissimus dorsi
• obliquus internus
• obliquus externus
• quadratus lumborum
• erector spinae
• multifidus spinae
• tractus iliotibialis
• gluteus maximus
• gluteus medius
• piriformis

❸ Keeping your hips aligned, rotate your upper spine as you pull your chest in toward your knee.

❹ Hold for thirty seconds. Slowly release, and repeat three times on each side.

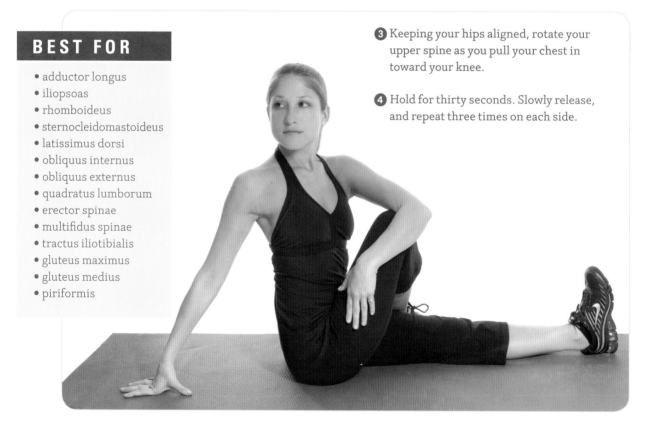

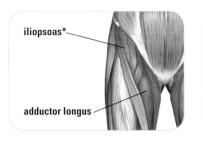

iliopsoas*

adductor longus

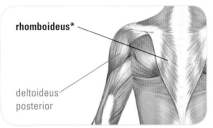

rhomboideus*

deltoideus posterior

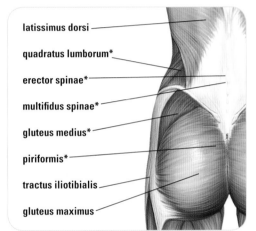

latissimus dorsi

quadratus lumborum*

erector spinae*

multifidus spinae*

gluteus medius*

piriformis*

tractus iliotibialis

gluteus maximus

QUICK GUIDE

TARGET
- Hips
- Gluteal muscles
- Spine
- Obliques

TYPE
- Flexibility

LEVEL
- Intermediate

BENEFITS
- Stretches hip extensors and flexors
- Stretches obliques

NOT ADVISABLE IF YOU HAVE
- Severe lower-back pain

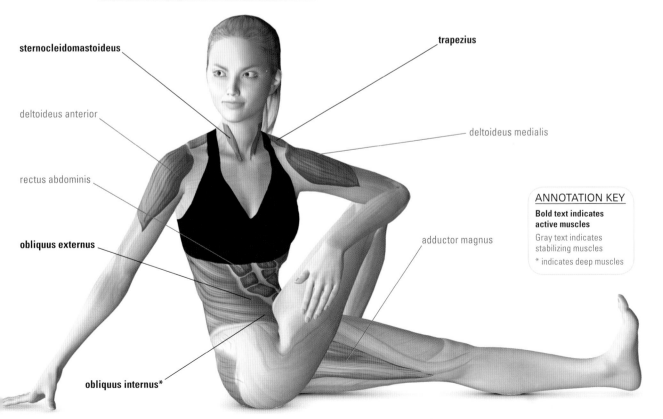

sternocleidomastoideus

trapezius

deltoideus anterior

deltoideus medialis

rectus abdominis

obliquus externus

adductor magnus

obliquus internus*

ANNOTATION KEY
Bold text indicates active muscles
Gray text indicates stabilizing muscles
* indicates deep muscles

SAMPLE WORKOUTS

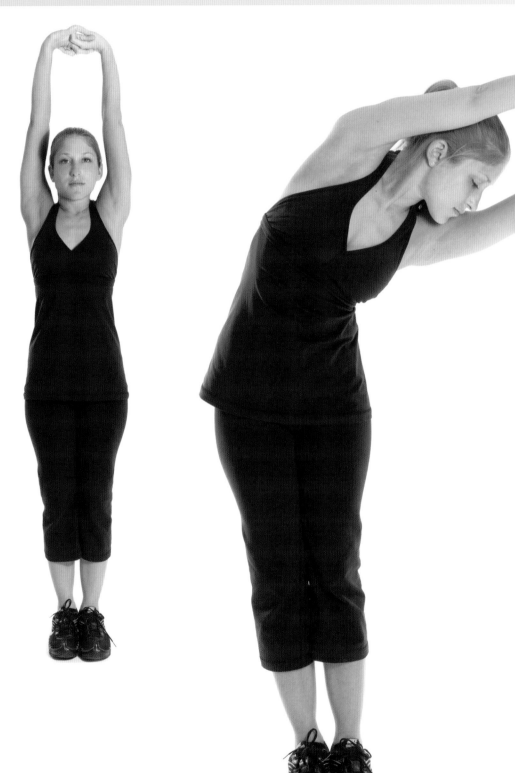

Now that you've familiarized yourself with a wide variety of healthy back exercises, it's time to put them to use. Included here is a basic cervical/thoracic routine, which will help work your neck and upper back. Following are two versions of a progressive lumbar/core workout. The first is designed to alleviate pain associated with forward movements of the lumbar spine, and the second targets those who experience pain when extending. The last sample workout combines exercises from all areas to stabilize and build your muscles. These sample workouts will help you get started on a consistent exercise routine, but you can create many additional combinations using the book's exercises. Remember to start slowly, taking into consideration your overall health and fitness level. Then have fun and mix things up once you feel comfortable with your routine.

CERVICAL/THORACIC

SAMPLE WORKOUTS

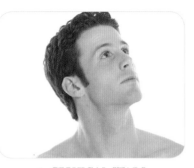

1. CERVICAL STARS
Page 34

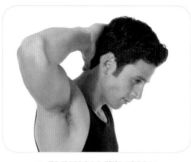

2. FLEXION STRETCH
Page 22

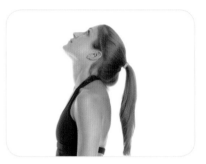

3. EXTENSION STRETCH
Page 28

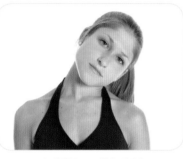

4. LATERAL STRETCH
Page 24

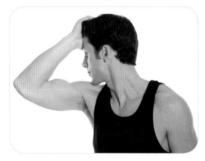

5. ROTATION STRETCH
Page 26

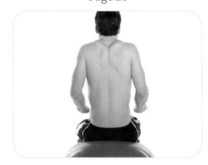

6. SHRUG
Page 32

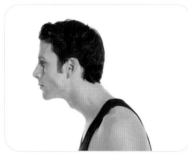

7. TURTLE NECK
Page 33

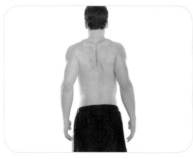

8. SCAPULAR RANGE OF MOTION
Page 38

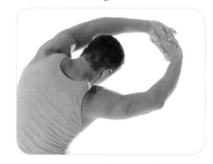

9. SIDE BENDING
Page 42

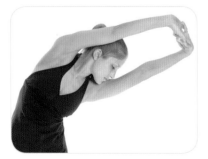

10. LATISSIMUS DORSI STRETCH
Page 44

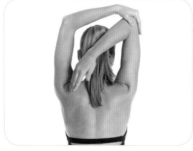

11. SHOULDER STRETCH I
Page 40

OR

SHOULDER STRETCH II
Page 41

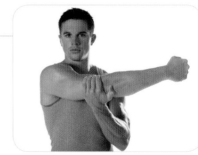

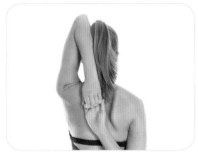

12. POSTERIOR HAND CLASP
Page 50

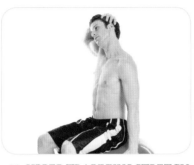

13. UPPER TRAPEZIUS STRETCH
Page 30

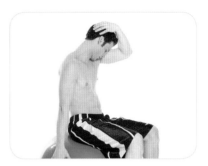

14. LEVATOR SCAPULAE STRETCH
Page 31

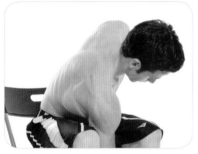

15. CHAIR TWIST
Page 48

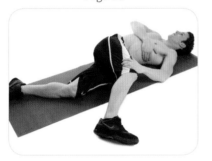

16. OPEN BOOK STRETCH
Page 47

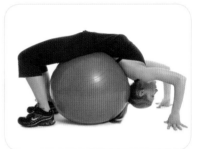

17. BACKWARD BALL STRETCH
Page 62

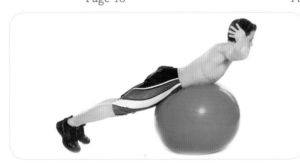

18. BODY BALL EXTENSION
Page 60

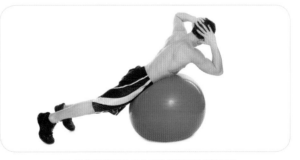

19. ROTATED BACK EXTENSION
Page 102

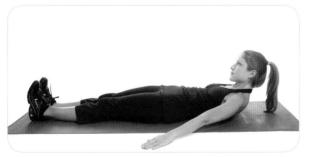

20. LOW CURL-UP
Page 82

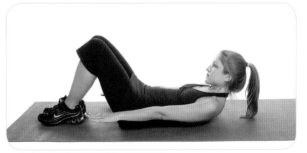

21. HALF CURL
Page 74

PROGRESSIVE LUMBAR/CORE

SAMPLE WORKOUTS

❶ FLEXION EXERCISES FOR PAINFUL EXTENSION

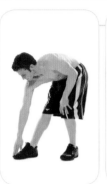 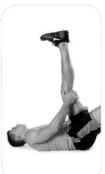

1.
HAMSTRING
STRETCH I
Page 140

OR

HAMSTRING
STRETCH II
Page 141

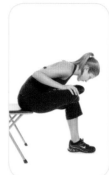 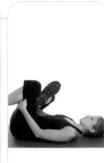

2.
SEATED
PIRIFORMIS
STRETCH
Page 78

OR

PIRIFORMIS
STRETCH
Page 79

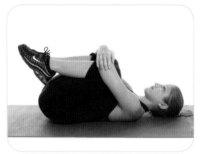 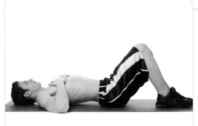 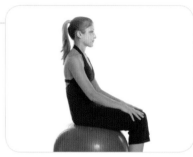

3. KNEE-TO-CHEST HUG
Page 119 (modification)

4. SUPINE PELVIC TILT
Page 114

OR

SEATED PELVIC TILT
Page 115

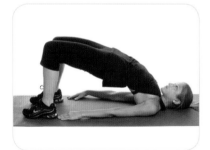 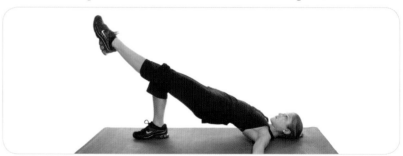

5. BRIDGE
Page 130

6. BRIDGE WITH LEG LIFT
Page 132

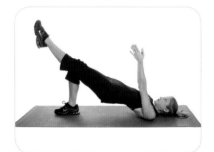 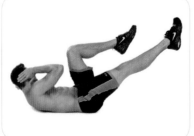 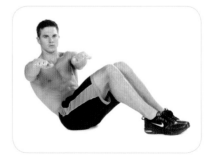

7. BRIDGE WITH LEG LIFT
Page 133 (modification)

8. CROSSOVER CRUNCH
Page 106

9. RUSSIAN TWIST
Page 80

❷ EXTENSION EXERCISES FOR PAINFUL FLEXION

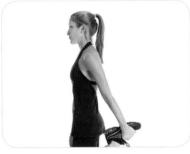

1. QUADRICEPS STRETCH
Page 136

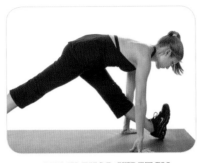

2. HIP FLEXOR STRETCH
Page 144

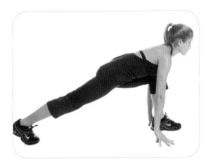

3. FORWARD LUNGE
Page 142

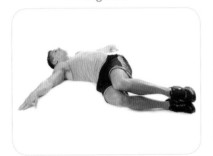

4. LOWER-BACK ROTATION
Page 121

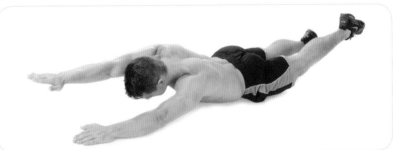

5. SWIMMING
Page 128

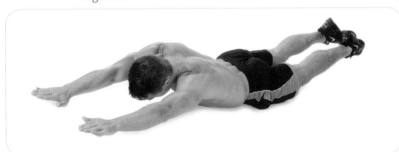

6. SWIMMING
Page 129 (Superman modification)

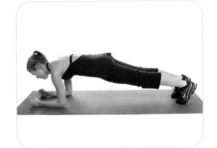

7. PLANK
Page 94

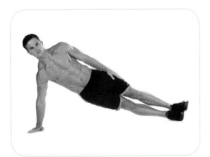

8. SIDE-BEND PLANK
Page 110

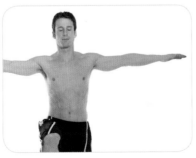

9. STANDING STABILITY
Page 68

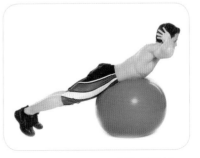

10. BODY BALL EXTENSION
Page 60

HEALTHY SPINE STABILIZATION

SAMPLE WORKOUTS

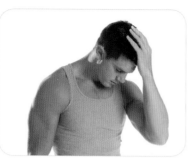

1. FLEXION ISOMETRIC
Page 23

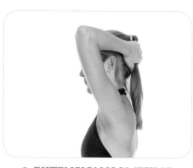

2. EXTENSION ISOMETRIC
Page 29

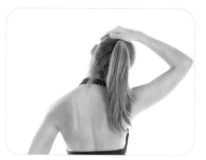

3. LATERAL ISOMETRIC
Page 25

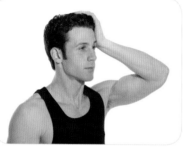

4. ROTATION ISOMETRIC
Page 27

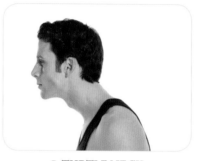

5. TURTLE NECK
Page 33

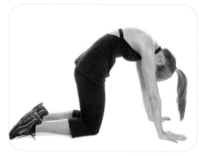

6. CAT AND DOG STRETCH
Page 124

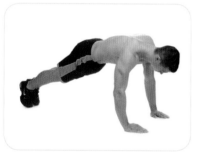

7. PLANK ROLL-DOWN
Page 90

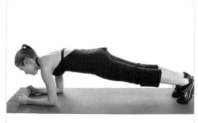

8. PLANK
Page 94

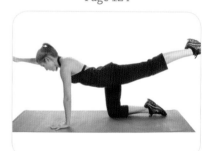

9. THE POINTER
Page 92

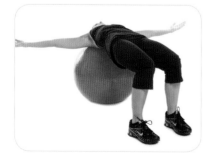

10. SIDE WALKING
Page 98

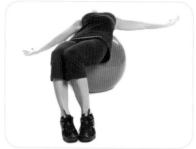

11. REVERSE BRIDGE BALL ROLL
Page 86

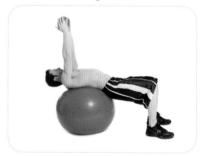

12. MEDICINE BALL AB CURLS
Page 88

& MUSCLE BUILDING

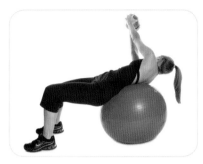

13. REVERSE BRIDGE ROTATION
Page 84

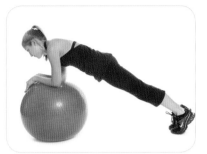

14. TRANSVERSE ABS
Page 104

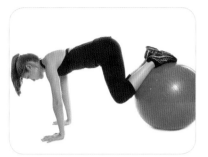

15. JACKKNIFE
Page 100

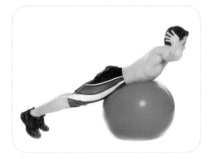

16. BODY BALL EXTENSION
Page 60

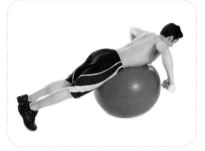

17. SWISS BALL ROW
Page 58

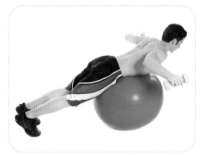

18. SWISS BALL REVERSE FLY
Page 56

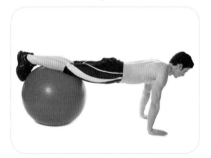

19. HAND WALKOUT
Page 52

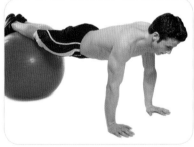

20. HAND WALK-AROUND
Page 54

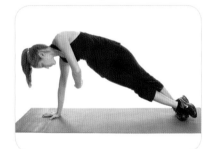

21. THE TWIST
Page 108

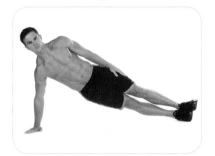

22. SIDE-BEND PLANK
Page 110

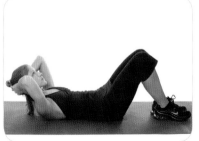

23. BASIC CRUNCH
Page 70

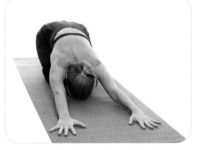

24. CHILD'S POSE
Page 122

GLOSSARY

GENERAL TERMS

abduction: Movement away from the body.

adduction: Movement toward the body.

alternating grip: One hand grasping with the palm facing toward the body and the other facing away.

anterior: Located in the front.

biomechanics: The sport science field that applies the laws of mechanics and physics to human performance.

cardiovascular exercise: Any exercise that increases the heart rate, making oxygen and nutrient-rich blood available to working muscles.

cardiovascular system: The circulatory system that distributes blood throughout the body, which includes the heart, lungs, arteries, veins, and capillaries.

cervical: Of, or relating to, the neck. The cervical vertebrae are the seven immediately inferior to the skull.

coccygeal: Referring to the coccyx. See *coccyx*.

coccyx: The small tail-like bone at the bottom of the spine.

concentric (contraction): Occurs when a muscle shortens in length and develops tension, e.g., the upward movement of a weight in a biceps curl.

crossed syndrome: Describes a compromise in the musculoskeletal system, which tightens, or facilitates, the anterior of one area of the body while at the same time weakening, or inhibiting, the posterior, usually resulting from a predictable pattern of muscular compensation and postural imbalances in the body. The "upper crossed syndrome" refers to imbalances in the upper torso, and the "lower crossed syndrome" refers to imbalances in the lower torso and legs. These syndromes were first described by Czech physiotherapist Dr. Vladimir Janda.

crunch: A common abdominal exercise that calls for curling the shoulders toward the pelvis while lying supine with hands behind head and knees bent.

curl: An exercise movement, usually targeting the biceps brachii, that calls for a weight to be moved through an arc, in a "curling" motion.

eccentric (contraction): The development of tension while a muscle is being lengthened, e.g., the downward movement of a weight in a biceps curl.

ergonomics: The study of designing equipment and devices that fit the human body, its movements, and its cognitive abilities.

extension: The act of straightening.

extensor muscle: A muscle serving to extend a body part away from the body.

facet joint: The joint between the articular processes of the vertebrae. Also called the zygapophyseal joint.

facilitated: Tightened, as in a muscle. See *crossed syndrome*.

flexion: The bending of a joint.

flexor muscle: A muscle that decreases the angle between two bones, as bending the arm at the elbow or raising the thigh toward the stomach.

fly: An exercise movement in which the hand and arm move through an arc while the elbow is kept at a constant angle.

iliotibial band (ITB): A thick band of fibrous tissue that runs down the outside of the leg, beginning at the hip and extending to the outer side of the tibia just below the knee joint. This band functions in coordination with several of the thigh muscles to provide stability to the outside of the knee joint.

inhibited: Weakened, as in a muscle. See *crossed syndrome*.

intervertebral disk: The layer of fibrocartilage between the bodies of adjoining vertebrae.

isometric exercise: A form of exercise involving the static contraction of a muscle without any visible movement in the angle of the joint.

kyphosis: The outward curvature of the spine; excessive kyphosis causes a humped back.

lateral: Located on, or extending toward, the outside.

ligament: The fibrous tissue that connects bones to other bones.

lordosis: The inward curvature of the spine; excessive lordosis causes a swayback.

lumbar: Of, near, or situated in the part of the back and sides between the lowest ribs and the pelvis; the lumbar vertebrae are the five vertebrae at the base of the spinal column.

medial: Located on, or extending toward, the middle.

medicine ball: A weighted ball, often used for rehabilitation and strength training.

muscle: The contractile tissue of the body that functions to produce force and cause motion. Cardiac and smooth muscle contraction occurs without conscious thought, and voluntary muscles, which we use to move the body, can be finely controlled.

nerve: A cordlike structure comprising a collection of fibers that convey impulses between a part of the central nervous system and some other body region.

nervous system: The system of cells, tissues, and organs that regulates the body's responses to internal and external stimuli. In humans, it consists of the brain, spinal cord, nerves, ganglia, and parts of the receptor and effector organs. The central nervous system is made up of the brain and spinal cord.

neural foramen: The aperture formed between every pair of vertebrae, which allows for the passage of the spinal column.

neutral position: A spinal position resembling an S shape, consisting of a lordosis in the lower back when viewed in profile.

overhand grip: A grip in which your palms are facing down and away from you, and your thumbs are pointing inward to each other. Also called a pronated grip.

physiatrist: A physician specializing in physical medicine and rehabilitation.

posterior: Located behind.

process: A prominence or projection, as from a bone. The spinous process of the vertebrae projects backward from the arches, giving attachment to the back muscles; the transverse processes project on either side of the arch of a vertebra.

pronated grip: See *overhand grip*.

sacral: Referring to the sacrum. See *sacrum*.

sacrum: The large heavy bone at the base of the spine, which is made up of fused sacral vertebrae. The lumbar vertebrae stack immediately on top of the sacrum.

scapula: The protrusion of bone on the mid to upper back, also known as the shoulder blade.

spinal column: The series of articulated vertebrae, separated by intervertebral disks and held together by muscles and tendons, that extends from the cranium to the coccyx, encasing the spinal cord and forming the supporting axis of the body. Also called the backbone, rachis, vertebral column, or spine.

spinal cord: The major column of nerve tissue that is connected to the brain and lies within the vertebral canal and from which the spinal nerves emerge. Thirty-one pairs of spinal nerves originate in the spinal cord: eight cervical, twelve thoracic, five lumbar, five sacral, and five coccygeal.

sternum: The elongated, flattened bone forming the middle portion of the anterior wall of the thorax. Its upper end supports the clavicles, or collarbones, and its margins articulate with the cartilages of the first seven pairs of ribs.

Swiss ball: A flexile, inflatable PVC ball measuring approximately 14 to 34 inches in circumference that is used for weight training, physical therapy, balance training, and other exercise regimens. It is also called a stability ball, fitness ball, exercise ball, gym ball, physioball, and many other names.

tendon: A tough band of fibrous connective tissue that usually connects muscle to bone.

thoracic: Of, relating to, or situated in or near the thorax; the thoracic vertebrae are the twelve between the cervical vertebrae and the lumbar vertebrae.

thorax: The region of the body formed by the sternum, the thoracic vertebrae, and the ribs, extending from the neck to the diaphragm, and not including the upper limbs.

vertebra: The bones that make up the spine.

vertebral body: The weight-supporting, solid central part of a vertebra.

vertebral canal: The canal formed within the spinal column that contains the spinal cord.

vestibular deficit: Difficulties maintaining balance due to inner-ear disorders.

warm-up: Any form of light exercise of short duration that prepares the body for more intense exercises.

zygapophyseal joint: See *facet joint*.

GLOSSARY

GLOSSARY

LATIN TERMS

The following glossary explains the Latin terminology used to describe the body's muscles, ligaments, and bones. Certain words are derived from Greek or French, which has been indicated in each instance.

CHEST

coracobrachialis: Greek *korakoeidés*, "ravenlike," and *brachium*, "arm"

costae: *costa*, "rib"

pectoralis (major and minor): *pectus*, "breast"

ABDOMEN

obliquus externus: *obliquus*, "slanting," and *externus*, "outward"

obliquus internus: *obliquus*, "slanting," and *internus*, "within"

rectus abdominis: *rego*, "straight, upright," and *abdomen*, "belly"

serratus anterior: *serra*, "saw," and *ante*, "before"

transversus abdominis: *transversus*, "athwart," and *abdomen*, "belly"

NECK

longus capitis: *longus*, "tall," and *capitis*, "of a head"

longus colli: *longus*, "tall," and *collum*, "neck"

rectus capitis: *rego*, "straight, upright," and *capitis*, "of a head"

rectus capitis lateralis: *rego*, "straight, upright," *capitis*, "of a head," and *lateralis*, "side"

scalenus: Greek *skalénós*, "unequal"

semispinalis: *semi*, "half," and *spinae*, "spine"

splenius: Greek *splénion*, "plaster, patch"

sternocleidomastoideus: Greek *stérnon*, "chest," Greek *kleís*, "key," and Greek *mastoeidés*, "breastlike"

sternohyoideus: Greek *stérnon*, "chest," and Greek *hyoeides*, "U-shaped"

BACK

articulationes zygapophysiales: *articulatio*, "joint," Greek *zygo*, "yoke," and Greek *apophyses*, "an outgrowth or swelling"

erector spinae: *erectus*, "straight," and *spina*, "thorn"

latissimus dorsi: *latus*, "wide," and *dorsum*, "back"

multifidus spinae: *multifid*, "to cut into divisions," and *spinae*, "spine"

quadratus lumborum: *quadratus*, "square, rectangular," and *lumbus*, "loin"

rhomboideus: Greek *rhembesthai*, "to spin"

trapezius: Greek *trapezion*, "small table"

SHOULDERS

deltoideus (anterior, medial, and posterior): Greek *deltoeidés*, "delta-shaped"

infraspinatus: *infra*, "under," and *spina*, "thorn"

levator scapulae: *levare*, "to raise," and *scapulae*, "shoulder [blades]"

scapula: *scapulae*, "shoulder [blades]"

subscapularis: *sub*, "below," and *scapulae*, "shoulder [blades]"

supraspinatus: *supra*, "above," and *spina*, "thorn"

teres (major and minor): *teres*, "rounded"

UPPER ARM

biceps brachii: *biceps*, "two-headed," and *brachium*, "arm"

brachialis: *brachium*, "arm"

triceps brachii: *triceps*, "three-headed," and *brachium*, "arm"

LOWER ARM

anconeus: Greek *anconad*, "elbow"

brachioradialis: *brachium*, "arm," and *radius*, "spoke"

extensor carpi radialis: *extendere*, "to extend," Greek *karpós*, "wrist," and *radius*, "spoke"

extensor digitorum: *extendere*, "to extend," and *digitus*, "finger, toe"

flexor carpi pollicis longus: *flectere*, "to bend," Greek *karpós*, "wrist," *pollicis*, "thumb," and *longus*, "long"

flexor carpi radialis: *flectere*, "to bend," Greek *karpós*, "wrist," and *radius*, "spoke"

flexor carpi ulnaris: *flectere*, "to bend," Greek *karpós*, "wrist," and *ulnaris*, "forearm"

flexor digitorum: *flectere*, "to bend," and *digitus*, "finger, toe"

palmaris longus: *palmaris*, "palm," and *longus*, "long"

pronator teres: *pronate*, "to rotate," and *teres*, "rounded"

HIPS

gemellus (inferior and superior): *geminus*, "twin"

gluteus maximus: Greek *gloutós*, "rump," and *maximus*, "largest"

gluteus medius: Greek *gloutós*, "rump," and *medialis*, "middle"

gluteus minimus: Greek *gloutós*, "rump," and *minimus*, "smallest"

iliacus: *ilium*, "groin"

iliopsoas: *ilium*, "groin," and Greek *psoa*, "groin muscle"

obturator externus: *obturare*, "to block," and *externus*, "outward"

obturator internus: *obturare*, "to block," and *internus*, "within"

pectineus: *pectin*, "comb"

piriformis: *pirum*, "pear," and *forma*, "shape"

quadratus femoris: *quadratus*, "square, rectangular," and *femur*, "thigh"

UPPER LEG

adductor longus: *adducere*, "to contract," and *longus*, "long"

adductor magnus: *adducere*, "to contract," and *magnus*, "major"

biceps femoris: *biceps*, "two-headed," and *femur*, "thigh"

gracilis: *gracilis*, "slim, slender"

rectus femoris: *rego*, "straight, upright," and *femur*, "thigh"

sartorius: *sarcio*, "to patch" or "to repair"

semimembranosus: *semi*, "half," and *membrum*, "limb"

semitendinosus: *semi*, "half," and *tendo*, "tendon"

tensor fasciae latae: *tenere*, "to stretch," *fasciae*, "band," and *latae*, "laid down"

vastus intermedius: *vastus*, "immense, huge," and *intermedius*, "between"

vastus lateralis: *vastus*, "immense, huge," and *lateralis*, "side"

vastus medialis: *vastus*, "immense, huge," and *medialis*, "middle"

LOWER LEG

adductor digiti minimi: *adducere*, "to contract," *digitus*, "finger, toe," and *minimum,* "smallest"

adductor hallucis: *adducere*, "to contract," and *hallex*, "big toe"

extensor digitorum: *extendere*, "to extend," and *digitus*, "finger, toe"

extensor hallucis: *extendere*, "to extend," and *hallex*, "big toe"

flexor digitorum: *flectere*, "to bend," and *digitus*, "finger, toe"

flexor hallucis: *flectere*, "to bend," and *hallex*, "big toe"

gastrocnemius: Greek *gastroknémía*, "calf [of the leg]"

peroneus: *peronei*, "of the fibula"

plantaris: *planta*, "sole"

soleus: *solea*, "sandal"

tibialis anterior: *tibia*, "reed pipe," and *ante*, "before"

tibialis posterior: *tibia*, "reed pipe," and *posterus*, "coming after"

trochlea tali: *trochleae*, "a pulley-shaped structure," and *talus*, "lower portion of ankle joint"

LIGAMENTS

ligamentum capsular facet: *ligamentum*, "bandage," *capsa*, "box," and *facies*, "face"

ligamentum interspinalis: *ligamentum*, "bandage," *inter*, "between," and *spina*, "thorn"

ligamentum longitudinale anterius: *ligamentum*, "bandage," *longitudo*, "length," and *ante*, "in front"

ligamentum longitudinale posterius: *ligamentum*, "bandage," *longitudo*, "length," and *post*, "behind"

ligamentum nuchae: *ligamentum*, "bandage," and French *nuque*, "nape"

ligamentum supraspinous: *ligamentum*, "bandage," *supra*, "above," and *spina*, "thorn"

ligamentum transversum: *ligamentum*, "bandage" and *transversus*, "athwart"

CREDITS & ACKNOWLEDGMENTS

All photographs by Jonathan Conklin/Jonathan Conklin Photography, Inc., except page 14 by grafvision/Shutterstock and page 16 by Simon Krzic/Shutterstock

Poster illustrations by Linda Bucklin/Shutterstock

Models: Goldie Karpel, Michael Galizia, and Michael Radon

All anatomical illustrations by Hector Aiza/3D Labz Animation India, except the insets on pages 22, 23, 24, 26, 27, 28, 29, 43, 45, 46, 47, 49, 51, 53, 55, 57, 59, 61, 63, 67, 68, 69, 71, 77, 79, 85, 87, 89, 95, 101, 103, 105, 111, 114, 117, 119, 120, 121, 123, 125, 127, 131, 133, 139, 140, 145, and 147 by Linda Bucklin/Shutterstock and pages 41 and 97 by 3D4Medical; and the illustrations on pages 8 and 15 by Alex Mit/Shutterstock; page 9 by Sebastian Kaulitzkin/Shutterstock; page 10 by BioMedical/Shutterstock; page 17 by Patrick Hermans/Shutterstock, and pages 18 and 19 by Linda Bucklin/Shutterstock

ACKNOWLEDGMENTS

Since 1994, I have had the distinct privilege of treating thousands of individuals from many different walks of life. Healing people and helping them return to the activities of their lives—from grandparents playing with their grandchildren to athletes getting back on the field to workers returning to their jobs—has been incredibly rewarding for me.

I want to take this opportunity to thank my parents, Drs. Philip and Theresa Striano, for guiding me through the years to get to this point in my life. Dad, although my time with you was short, your sacrifice and conviction for your profession, patients, and family will always be a guiding force for me. I also want to acknowledge my three sisters, Terri, Thomasina, and Tara, for the their love and support.

My two boys, Christian and Brandon, you two fill my life with joy and pride— I love you both with all my heart! Shelly and Stacy, thank you both for these two divine gifts.

I firmly believe that all people become who they are through their interpersonal interactions with others. I would like to thank some of these people, who throughout my life, have made me the person I am today: from Hackley School, the Stern, Allen, Khosrowshahi, Leary, and Chervokas families; from the Franklin and Marshall football and lacrosse team, my teammates; and from ACC, the Lifflanders, Pilzers, and Proshop.

Thanks to Dr. Richard Brodsky for helping with the book. Thanks to Cheech for being Cheech.

Finally, thanks to Lisa, Sean, and Karen for giving me this opportunity!

The author and publisher also offer thanks to those closely involved in the creation of this book: Moseley Road president Sean Moore; editorial director/designer Lisa Purcell; general manager Karen Prince; art director Brian MacMullen; designers Hwaim Holly Lee and Katie Calak; and editorial assistant Rebecca Axelrad.